KT-150-947

'Brilliantly detailed and wholly convincing: with Coyle's skill and Hamilton's honesty, the book was always likely to be excellent. This is no generalised or theoretical exploration of a doping culture but a forensic description of how it worked. Armstrong used to say there would always be sceptics who didn't believe in his story, but now the sceptics are those who, ostrich-like, continue to believe. They should be compelled to read this book, and though the collision with reality will cause them to shudder, the good news is that they will be riveted by a well-told story and will be the better for knowing the truth'
David Walsh, *Sunday Times*

'The broadest, most accessible look at cycling's drug problem to date'
New York Times

'The news leaks about *The Secret Race* have vastly undersold its importance. Tyler Hamilton's book is a historic, definitive indictment of cycling's culture of doping during the Armstrong era. Here's the reality. *The Secret Race* isn't just a game changer for the Armstrong myth. It's the game ender. No one can read this book with an open mind and still credibly believe that Armstrong didn't dope. It's impossible. That doesn't change the fact that he survived cancer and helped millions of people through Livestrong, but the myth of the clean-racing hero who came back from the dead is, well, dead. The book is the holy grail for disillusioned cycling fans in search of answers. The book's power is in the collected details, all strung together in a story that is told with such clear-eyed conviction that you never doubt its veracity'
Outside magazine

'Astonishingly candid . . . an extraordinary confessional'
Matt Dickinson, *The Times*

'Riveting . . . Just about every significant detail in the USADA evidence is here. And it is brilliantly conveyed by an insider who can see both sides of the story: the institutional corruption, which eats away at the culprits, as well as the crippling pressure on riders to conform. We can expect plenty more books to be published on this

conspiracy, for it is arguably the most audacious ever plotted in the world of sport. But it feels as though Hamilton's is likely to become the definitive work on the subject'
Simon Briggs, *Daily Telegraph*

'The book that finally broke Lance Armstrong'
Sport magazine

'The mysterious world of cycling holds a certain fascination in the public consciousness – now more than ever following the recent home-grown success in the sport. *The Secret Race* lifts the lid on that world and delivers a shocking and jaw-droppingly frank account of what it's like to compete at the highest level'
Graham Sharpe, William Hill Sports Book of the Year

'A landmark publication . . . absolutely brilliant. *The Secret Race* stood out because it fundamentally changed the sport it described. I wish it hadn't had to be written, but it is a book that has to be read'
John Inverdale

'The insight into the sporting mindset is uncanny; the detail unforgettable. A gruesomely compelling instant classic'
Sunday Telegraph, Sports Books of the Year

'The book inspired in me not surprise so much as the occasional jolt of shock at the grimy practicalities and the odd drop of my jaw at the means Hamilton says that he, Lance Armstrong and others used to stay ahead of the testers and the police . . . A deep insight into the evidence that Armstrong refused to confront when he opted out of arbitration in the case that the US Anti-Doping Agency had built against him and his associates'
William Fotheringham, *Observer*

'Eye-popping revelations . . . The strength of Hamilton's testimony lies in the forensic detail with which he describes how the doping system operated and how riders managed to cheat the testers for so long'
Simon Redfern, *Independent on Sunday*

'A searingly honest piece of work, a forensic and hugely important study of how a sport turned rotten'
Tom English, *Scotland on Sunday*

'Brilliant . . . Daniel Coyle and Tyler Hamilton finally lay bare an awful truth and back it up with hard forensic evidence. The result is a book of searing honesty, the clearest possible description of what had been going on behind the scenes at many pro cycling teams for decades. *The Secret Race* draws the curtain back on cycling's cheating and corruption with admirable ferocity'
Burton Mail

'Gripping . . . extraordinary'
David Runciman, *London Review of Books*

'I wasn't expecting to be moved by Hamilton's book. He broke my heart in 2004 and he's a self-confessed cheat after all. But it is an honest, harrowing, eye-opening account that is a must-read for anyone interested in competitive cycling in the late '90s and the early 2000s. I came away with a better appreciation of the professional cyclist, under pressure to succeed. I came away with a renewed respect for Tyler Hamilton despite his misdemeanours. But most surprisingly of all, I came away with a renewed love of the sport. For underneath all the talk about things he did wrong - and he points the finger at himself more than any other - there runs a passionate dialogue about cycling. A sport that defines him. A sport that ruined him. But ultimately, a sport that is all the better for Tyler Hamilton's candid portrayal of life in the peloton'
Julia Stagg, *Freewheeling France*

'A valuable document and a well-timed one'
Gary Imlach, *New Statesman*

'A gripping tale'
Chris Maume, *Independent*, Books of the Year 2012

'2012 was the year in which a handful of books changed what we thought we knew about the games we love to watch and play. None more so than the recent William Hill Sports Book of the Year, *The Secret Race*. Cyclist Tyler Hamilton's confessional of his time on Lance Armstrong's US Postal Service Team, written with Daniel Coyle, is a fascinating insight. It revealed in such incredible detail the culture of systematic doping, in which Hamilton took part, that the whole sport was changed forever. Within a month of its publication, combined with the damning USADA report, Armstrong had been stripped of his Tour de France titles'
Ben East, *Metro*, Books of the Year

'A courageous act of witness'
The Economist

'An obvious choice, ultimately. A book that went beyond entertainment or education in their normal senses. This is the book that opened the world's eyes to the incredible doping scandal in cycling and the crimes of Lance Armstrong. A book that will be on almost all awards lists for books this year, and will surely migrate to the lists of all-time great books as its impact becomes more apparent over time'
Newstalk, Sports Book of the Year

'Explosive . . . a stunning and sometimes sickening account of the doping pervasive in the pro peloton'
Sports Illustrated

'Haunting . . . takes readers deep inside the gory cult of back-alley phlebotomy that ruled cycling as Armstrong launched and nurtured his Livestrong brand'
New York Daily News

THE SECRET RACE

INSIDE THE HIDDEN WORLD OF THE TOUR DE FRANCE: DOPING, COVER-UPS, AND WINNING AT ALL COSTS

Tyler Hamilton
and
Daniel Coyle

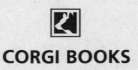

CORGI BOOKS

TRANSWORLD PUBLISHERS
61–63 Uxbridge Road, London W5 5SA
A Random House Group Company
www.transworldbooks.co.uk

THE SECRET RACE
A CORGI BOOK: 9780552169172

First published in Great Britain
in 2012 by Bantam Press
an imprint of Transworld Publishers
Corgi edition published 2013

Copyright© Tyler Hamilton and Daniel Coyle 2012
Afterword © Tyler Hamilton and Daniel Coyle 2013

Tyler Hamilton and Daniel Coyle have asserted their right under the Copyright,
Designs and Patents Act 1988 to be identified as the authors of this work.

Book design by Christopher M. Zucker.

A CIP catalogue record for this book
is available from the British Library.

This book is sold subject to the condition that it shall not,
by way of trade or otherwise, be lent, resold, hired out,
or otherwise circulated without the publisher's prior
consent in any form of binding or cover other than that
in which it is published and without a similar condition,
including this condition, being imposed on the
subsequent purchaser.

Addresses for Random House Group Ltd companies outside the UK
can be found at: www.randomhouse.co.uk
The Random House Group Ltd Reg. No. 954009

The Random House Group Limited supports The Forest Stewardship Council®
(FSC®), the leading international forest-certification organisation. Our books
carrying the FSC label are printed on FSC®-certified paper. FSC is the only
forest-certification scheme supported by the leading environmental organisations,
including Greenpeace. Our paper-procurement policy can be found at
www.randomhouse.co.uk/environment

Typeset in 12/14.5pt Bembo by Falcon Oast Graphic Art Ltd.
Printed and bound by CPI Group (UK) Ltd, Croydon, CR0 4YY.

8 10 9 7

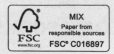

To my mom. — TH

To Jen. — DC

If you shut up the truth and bury it under the ground, it will but grow and gather to itself such explosive power that the day it bursts through it will blow up everything in its way.

—*Émile Zola*

Contents

THE SECRET RACE

THE STORY BEHIND THIS BOOK

Daniel Coyle

IN 2004, I MOVED TO SPAIN with my family to write a book about Lance Armstrong's attempt to win his sixth Tour de France. It was a fascinating project for many reasons, the biggest being the mystery glowing at its center: Who was Lance Armstrong, really? Was he a true and worthy champion, as many believed? Was he a doper and a cheat, as others insisted? Or did he live in the shadowy space in between?

We rented an apartment in Armstrong's training base of Girona, a ten-minute walk from the fortresslike home Armstrong shared with his then-girlfriend, Sheryl Crow. I lived fifteen months on Planet Lance, spending time with Armstrong's friends, teammates, doctors, coaches, lawyers, agents, mechanics, masseuses, rivals, detractors, and, of course, Armstrong himself.

I liked Armstrong's abundant energy, his sharp sense of humor, and his leadership abilities. I didn't like his volatility, secrecy, or the sometimes bullying way he would treat teammates and friends—but then again, this wasn't tiddly winks: it was the most physically and mentally demanding sport on the planet. I reported all sides of the story as thoroughly as I could, and then wrote *Lance Armstrong's War*, which several of Armstrong's teammates judged to be objective and fair. (Armstrong went on record as saying he was "okay" with the book.)

In the months and years after the book was published, people often asked me if I thought Armstrong doped. I was 50–50 on the question, with the likelihood rising steadily as time passed. On one hand, you had the circumstantial evidence: Studies showed dope boosted performance 10–15 percent in a sport where races were often decided by a fraction of a percentage point. You had the fact that almost every other rider who stood on the Tour de France podium with Armstrong was eventually linked to doping, along with five of Armstrong's U.S. Postal Service teammates. You had Armstrong's longtime close association with Dr. Michele (pronounced mi-KEL-ay) Ferrari, aka "Dr. Evil," the mysterious Italian acknowledged as one of the sport's most infamous doctors.

On the other hand, you had the fact that Armstrong had passed scores of drug tests with flying colors. You had the fact that he defended himself vigorously, and had prevailed in several high-profile lawsuits. Plus, in the back of my mind there was always the fallback reasoning: if it turned out that Armstrong *was* doping, then it was a level playing field, wasn't it?

Whatever the truth, I was 100 percent sure that I was never going to write about doping and/or Armstrong again. To put it simply, doping was a bummer. Sure, it was fascinating in a cloak-and-dagger sort of way, but the deeper you went, the nastier and murkier it got: stories of dangerously unqualified doctors, Machiavellian team directors, and desperately ambitious riders who suffered profound physical and psychological damage. It was dark stuff, made darker during my time in Girona by the deaths of two of the Armstrong era's brightest stars: Marco Pantani (depression, cocaine overdose, age thirty-four) and José María Jiménez (depression, heart attack, age thirty-two), and the suicide attempt of another star, thirty-year-old Frank Vandenbroucke.

Surrounding it all, like a vault of hardened steel, was the omertà: the rule of silence that governs professional racers when it comes to doping. The omertà's strength was well established: in the sport's long history, no top-level rider had ever revealed all. Support riders and team personnel who spoke about doping were cast out of the brotherhood and treated as traitors. With so little reliable information, reporting on doping was an exercise in frustration, especially when it came to Armstrong, whose iconic status as a cancer-fighting citizen saint both drew scrutiny and sheltered him from it. When *War* was finished, I moved on to other projects, content to see Planet Lance receding in my rearview mirror.

Then, in May 2010, everything changed.

The U.S. government opened a grand jury investigation into Armstrong and his U.S. Postal team. The lines of inquiry included fraud, conspiracy, racketeering, bribery of foreign officials, and witness intimidation. The investigation was led by federal prosecutor Doug Miller and investigator Jeff Novitzky, who'd played major roles in the Barry Bonds/BALCO case. That summer, they began to shine a bright spotlight into the darkest corners of Planet Lance. They subpoenaed witnesses—Armstrong teammates, staffers, and friends—to testify before a Los Angeles grand jury.

I began to receive calls. Sources told me that the investigation was big and getting bigger: that Novitzky had uncovered eyewitness evidence that Armstrong had transported, used, and distributed controlled substances, and evidence that he may have had access to experimental blood replacement drugs. As Dr. Michael Ashenden, an Australian anti-doping specialist who had worked on several major doping investigations, told me, "If Lance manages to get out of this one, he'll be bloody Houdini."

As the investigation progressed, I began to feel the tug of unfinished business, the sense that this might be an opportunity to discover the real story of the Armstrong era. The problem was, I couldn't report this story on my own. I needed a guide, someone who had lived in this world and was willing to break the omertà. There was really only one name to consider: Tyler Hamilton.

Tyler Hamilton was no saint. He had been one of the world's top-ranked, best-known racers, winner of the Olympic gold medal, until he was busted for doping in 2004 and exiled from the sport. His connection to Armstrong went back more than a decade, first as Armstrong's top lieutenant on U.S. Postal from 1998 to 2001, then as a rival when Hamilton left Postal to lead CSC and Phonak. The two also happened to be neighbors, living in the same Girona building, Armstrong on the second floor, Hamilton and his wife, Haven, on the third.

Before his fall, Hamilton had been regarded as the sort of Everyman hero sportswriters used to invent in the 1950s: soft-spoken, handsome, polite, and tough beyond conventional measure. He hailed from Marblehead, Massachusetts, where he had been a top downhill skier until college, when a back injury caused him to discover his true calling. Hamilton was the opposite of a flashy superstar: a blue-collar racer who slowly, patiently ascended the pyramid of the cycling world. Along the way, he became known for his unparalleled work ethic, his low-key, friendly personality, and, most of all, his remarkable ability to endure pain.

In 2002 Hamilton crashed early in the three-week Tour of Italy, fracturing his shoulder. He kept riding, enduring such pain that he ground eleven teeth down to the roots, requiring surgery after the Tour. He finished second. "In 48 years of practicing I have never seen a man who could handle as much pain as he can," said Hamilton's physical therapist, Ole Kare Foli.

In 2003 Hamilton performed an encore, crashing in stage 1 of the Tour de France and fracturing his collarbone. He kept going, winning a stage and finishing a remarkable fourth in a performance that veteran Tour doctor Gérard Porte described as "the finest example of courage I've come across."

Hamilton was also one of the better-liked riders in the peloton: humble, quick to praise others, and considerate. Hamilton's teammates enjoyed performing a skit in which one teammate would pretend to be Hamilton lying crumpled on the road after a crash. The other teammate, pretending to be the team doctor, would race up to Hamilton, distraught. "Oh my God, Tyler," he would shout, "your leg's been cut off! Are you okay?" The teammate playing Hamilton would smile reassuringly. "Oh, don't worry, I'm fine," he would say. "How are *you* feeling today?"

I'd spent time with Hamilton in Girona in 2004, and it had been a memorable experience. Most of the time, Hamilton was exactly as advertised: humble, nice, polite, every inch the Boy Scout. He opened the door for me, thanked me three times for buying the coffee; was charmingly ineffectual when it came to controlling his exuberant golden retriever, Tugboat. When we talked about life in Girona, or his childhood in Marblehead, or his beloved Red Sox, he was funny, perceptive, and engaged.

When he talked about bike racing or the upcoming Tour de France, however, Hamilton's personality changed. His playful sense of humor evaporated; his eyes locked onto his coffee cup, and he began to speak in the broadest, blandest, most boring sports clichés you've ever heard. He told me he was preparing for the Tour by "taking it one day, one race at a time, and doing his homework"; how Armstrong was "a great guy, a tough competitor, and a close friend"; how the Tour de France was "a real honor just to be a part of," etc., etc. It was as if he had a rare disorder that caused outbreaks of uncontrollable dullness whenever bike racing was mentioned.

In our last conversation (which happened a few weeks

before he was busted for blood doping), Hamilton had surprised me by asking if I might be interested in writing a book with him about his life in cycling. I'd said that I was flattered to be asked, and that we should talk about it more someday. To be honest, I was putting him off. As I told my wife that evening, I liked Hamilton, and his feats on the bike were amazing and inspiring, but when it came to being the subject of a book, he was fatally flawed: he was simply too boring.

A few weeks later, I found out that I had been mistaken. As news reports over the following months and years would reveal, the Boy Scout had been leading a second life straight out of a spy novel: code names, secret phones, tens of thousands of dollars in cash payments to a notorious Spanish doctor, and a medical freezer named "Siberia" for storing blood to be used at the Tour de France. Later, a Spanish police investigation revealed that Hamilton was far from alone: several dozen other top racers were on similarly elaborate secret programs. Against all evidence, Hamilton maintained he was innocent. His claims were rejected by anti-doping authorities; Hamilton was suspended for two years, and promptly dropped off the radar screen.

Now, as the Armstrong investigation accelerated, I did some research. The articles said Hamilton was nearing forty, divorced, and living in Boulder, Colorado, where he ran a small training and fitness business. He'd attempted a brief comeback after his suspension, which had ended when he tested positive for a non-performance-enhancing drug he'd taken to deal with his clinical depression, which he'd suffered from since he was a child. He wasn't giving interviews. A former teammate referred to Hamilton as "the Enigma."

I still had his email address. I wrote:

> *Hi Tyler,*
> *I hope this finds you well.*
> *A long time ago you asked me about writing a book together.*
> *If that's something that still appeals to you, I'd love to talk about it.*
>
> > *Best,*
> > *Dan*

A few weeks later, I flew to Denver to meet Hamilton. When I walked out of the terminal I saw him behind the wheel of a silver SUV. Hamilton's boyishness had weathered into something harder; his hair was longer and showed flecks of gray; the corners of his eyes held small, deep wrinkles. As we drove off, he cracked open a tin of chewing tobacco.

"I've been trying to quit. It's a filthy habit, I know. But with all the stress, it helps. Or at least it feels like it does."

We tried one restaurant, but Hamilton decided it was too crowded, and chose an emptier one down the block. Hamilton picked out a booth at the back, two candles burning on the table. He looked around. Then the man who could tolerate any pain—the one who'd ground his teeth down to the roots rather than quit—suddenly looked as if he was going to start crying. Not from grief, but from relief.

"Sorry," he said after a few seconds. "It just feels so

good to be able to talk about this, finally."

I started with the big question: Why had Hamilton lied before, about his own doping? Hamilton closed his eyes. He opened them again; I could see the sadness.

"Look, I lied. I thought it would cause the least damage. Put yourself in my shoes. If I had told the truth, everything's over. The team sponsor would pull out, and fifty people, fifty of my friends, would lose their jobs. People I care about. If I told the truth, I'd be out of the sport, forever. My name would be ruined. And you can't go partway—you can't just say, Oh, it was only me, just this one time. The truth is too big, it involves too many people. You've either got to tell 100 per-cent or nothing. There's no in-between. So yeah, I chose to lie. I'm not the first to do that, and I won't be the last. Sometimes if you lie enough you start to believe it."

Hamilton told me how, a few weeks before, he'd been subpoenaed by the investigation, placed under oath, and put on the stand in a Los Angeles courtroom.

"Before I went in I thought about it, a long time. I knew I couldn't lie to them, no way. So I decided that if I was going to tell the truth, I was going to go all the way. One hundred percent, full disclosure. I made up my mind that no question was going to stop me. That's what I did. I testified for seven hours. I answered everything they asked to the best of my ability. They kept asking me about Lance—they wanted me to point the finger at him. But I always pointed it at myself first. I made them understand how the whole system worked, got developed over the years, and how you couldn't single one person out. It was everybody. Everybody."

Hamilton rolled up his right and left sleeves. He put his palms up and extended his arms. He pointed to the crook of his elbows, to matching spidery scars that ran along his veins. "We all have scars like this," he said. "It's like a tattoo from a fraternity. When I got tan they'd show up and I'd have to lie about it; I'd tell people I cut my arm in a crash."

I asked how he avoided testing positive for all those years, and Hamilton gave a dry laugh.

"The tests are easy to beat," he said. "We're way, way ahead of the tests. They've got their doctors, and we've got ours, and ours are better. Better paid, for sure. Besides, the UCI [Union Cycliste Internationale, the sport's governing body] doesn't want to catch certain guys anyway. Why would they? It'd cost them money."

I asked why he wanted to tell his story now.

"I've been quiet for so many years," he said. "I buried it inside for so long. I've never really told it from beginning to end before, and so I'd never really seen it, or felt it. So once I started telling the truth, it was like this huge dam bursting inside me. And it feels so, so good to tell, I can't tell you how fantastic it feels. It felt like this giant weight is off my back, finally, and when I feel that, I know it's the right thing to do, for me and for the future of my sport."

The next morning, Hamilton and I met in my hotel room. I set out three ground rules.

1. No subject would be off limits.
2. Hamilton would give me access to his journals,

photos, and sources.

3. All facts would have to be independently confirmed whenever possible.

He agreed without hesitation.

That day, I interviewed Hamilton for eight hours—the first of more than sixty interviews. That December, we spent a week in Europe visiting key locations in Spain, France, and Monaco. To verify and corroborate Hamilton's account, I interviewed numerous independent sources—teammates, mechanics, doctors, spouses, team assistants, and friends—along with eight former U.S. Postal Service riders. Their accounts are also included in this book; some of them are coming forward for the first time.

Over the course of our relationship, I found Hamilton didn't tell his story so much as the story told him, emerging from him in extended bursts. He possesses an uncommonly precise memory, and proved accurate in his recollections, attributable, perhaps, to the emotional intensity of the original experiences. Hamilton's pain tolerance came in handy as well. He didn't spare himself in his process, encouraging me to talk with those who might hold him in an unfavorable light. In a way, he became as obsessed with revealing the truth as he was once obsessed with winning the Tour de France.

The interview process lasted nearly two years. At times I felt like a priest hearing a confession; at other times, like a shrink. As the time went by, I saw how telling gradually changed Hamilton. Our relationship turned out to be a journey for both of us. For Hamilton, it was a journey away from secrets and toward a normal life; for me, a trip toward the center of this never-before-seen world.

As it turned out, the story he told wasn't about doping; it was about power. It was about an ordinary guy who worked his way up to the top of an extraordinary world, who learned to play a shadowy chess match of strategy and information at the outermost edge of human performance. It was about a corrupt but strangely chivalrous world, where you would take any chemical under the sun to go faster, but wait for your opponent if he happened to crash. Above all, it was about the unbearable tension of living a secret life.

"One day I'm a normal person with a normal life," he said. "The next I'm standing on a street corner in Madrid with a secret phone and a hole in my arm and I'm bleeding all over, hoping I don't get arrested. It was completely crazy. But it seemed like the only way at the time."

Hamilton sometimes expressed fear that Armstrong and his powerful friends would act against him, but he never expressed any hatred for Armstrong. "I can feel for Lance," Hamilton said. "I understand who he is, and where he is. He made the same choice we all made, to become a player. Then he started winning the Tour and it got out of control, and the lies got bigger and bigger. Now he has no choice. He has to keep lying, to keep trying to convince people to move on. He can't go back. He can't tell the truth. He's trapped."

Armstrong did not respond to a request for an interview for this book. However, his legal representatives made it clear that he absolutely denies all doping allegations. As Armstrong said in a statement issued after the U.S. Anti-Doping Agency (USADA) charged him, his trainer, Dr. Ferrari, and four of his Postal team colleagues with doping conspiracy on June 12, 2012, "I have never doped, and, unlike many of my accusers, I have competed as an endurance athlete for 25 years with no spike in performance, passed more than 500 drug tests and never failed one."

Several of Armstrong's colleagues charged by USADA have also adamantly denied any involvement in doping activities, including former Postal director Johan Bruyneel, Dr. Luis del Moral, and Dr. Ferrari. In an interview with *The Wall Street Journal*, del Moral said he'd never provided banned drugs or performed illegal procedures on athletes. In a statement on his website, Bruyneel said, "I have never participated in any doping activity and I am innocent of all charges." In an emailed statement, Ferrari said, "I NEVER was found in possession of any EPO or testosterone in my life. I NEVER administrated EPO or testosterone to any athlete." Dr. Pedro Celaya and Pepe Martí, Dr. del Moral's assistant, who were also charged by USADA, made no public statements. The five did not respond to requests for interviews for this book. Bjarne Riis, who served as Hamilton's director on Team CSC from 2002 to 2003, offered the following statement: "I'm really saddened by these allegations that are being brought forward about me. But as this is not the first time someone is trying to miscredit me and, unfortunately, probably not the last time either, I will completely refrain from commenting on these allegations. I personally feel I deserve my spot in the world of cycling, and that I have made a contribution to strengthen the anti-doping work in the sport. I did my own confession to doping, I have been a key player in the creation of the biological passport, and I run a team with a clear anti-doping policy."

"The thing was, Lance was always different from the rest of us," Hamilton said. "We all wanted to win. But Lance *needed* to win. He had to make 100 percent sure that he won, every time, and that made him do some things that went way over the line, in my opinion. I understand that he's done a lot of good for a lot of people, but it still isn't right. Should he be prosecuted, go to prison for what he did? I don't think so. But should he have won seven Tours in a row? Absolutely not. So yes, I think people have the right to know the truth. People need to know how it all really happened, and then they can make up their own minds."*

---

* In the pages that follow, I'll be providing context and commentary to Hamilton's account through footnotes.

Chapter 1

GETTING IN THE GAME

I'M GOOD AT PAIN.

I know that sounds strange, but it's true. In every other area of life, I'm an average person. I'm not a brainiac. I don't have superhuman reflexes. I'm five-eight, 160 pounds soaking wet. If you met me on the street, I wouldn't stand out in the least. But in situations where things are pushed to the mental and physical edge, I've got a gift. I can keep going *no matter what*. The tougher things get, the better I do. I'm not masochistic about it, because I've got a method. Here's the secret: You can't block out the pain. You have to embrace it.

I think part of it comes from my family. Hamiltons are tough; we always have been. My ancestors were rebellious Scots from a warring clan; my grandfathers were adventurous types: skiers and outdoorsmen. Grandpa Carl was one of the first people to ski down Mount Washington; Grandpa Arthur crewed on a tramp freighter to South America. My mom and dad met backcountry skiing in Tuckerman's Ravine, the steepest, most dangerous run in the Northeast—their version of a quiet, romantic date, I suppose. My dad owned an office-supply shop near Marblehead, a seaside town of twenty thousand north of Boston. His business had its ups and downs—as Grandpa Arthur used to say, we went from eating steak to eating hamburger. But my dad always found a way to battle back. When I was little, he used to tell me that it's not the size of the dog in the fight; it's the size of the fight in the dog. I know it's a cliché, but it's one that I believed with all my heart; still do.

We lived in an old yellow saltbox house at 37 High Street in the middle-class part of town. I was the youngest of three, behind my brother, Geoff, and my sister, Jennifer. Twenty-plus kids lived within two blocks, all about the same age. It was the age before parenting was invented, so we roamed free, returning inside only for meals and sleep. It wasn't a childhood so much as a never-ending series of competitions: street hockey, sailing, and swimming in summer; sledding, skating, and skiing in winter. We got into a decent amount of mischief: sneaking on board the rich people's yachts and using them as clubhouses, slaloming Big Wheels down the steeps of Dunn's Lane, inventing a new sport called Walter Payton Hedge Jumping—basically, you pick the nicest house with the tallest hedge, and you dive over it like Walter Payton used to jump over the defensive line. When the owners come out, run like heck.

My parents didn't place many demands on us, except that we always tell the truth, no matter what. My dad once told me that if we ever had a family crest, it would contain only one word: HONESTY. It's how Dad ran his business, and how we ran our family. Even when we got in trouble—especially when we got in trouble—if we faced up to the truth, my parents wouldn't be mad.

That's one of the reasons why, for one special day every summer, our family had a tradition of hosting the Mountain Goat Invitational Crazy Croquet Tournament in our backyard. The Mountain Goat Invitational has only one rule—cheating is strongly encouraged. In fact, you can do anything short of picking up your opponent's ball and chucking it into the Atlantic (which, come to think of it, might have been done a few times). It was big fun—the winner was always disqualified for cheating, and our friends got to enjoy the joke: the sight of those famously honest Hamiltons cheating their heads off.

As a kid I was scrappy, always racing to keep up with the bigger guys. By the time I was ten, my list of injuries was pretty long: stitches, broken bones, burst appendix, sprains, and the like (the emergency-room nurses jokingly suggested my parents buy a punch card—ten visits, the eleventh is free). It was caused by usual stuff: falling off fences, jumping from bunk beds, getting knocked by a Chevy while riding bikes to school. But whenever I was banged up, Mom would be there to dab my scrapes with a warm washcloth, give me a bandage and a kiss, and boot me out the door.

Dad and I were close, but Mom and I had a special bond. She was a great athlete in her own right, and when I was small I used to want to imitate her. Early each morning she would do an exercise routine in our living room—fifteen minutes of Jack LaLanne-type calisthenics.

I'd wake up early and sneak downstairs so I could join her. We made quite a pair: a four-year-old and his mom doing push-ups and jumping jacks. *A*-one-*two-three-four,* two-*two-three-four.* . . .

That wasn't the only thing that made Mom and me close. For as long as I can remember, I've had this problem. The closest I can come to describing it is to say that it's a darkness that lives on the edge of my mind, a painful heaviness that comes and goes unexpectedly. When it comes on, it's like a black wave, pressing all the energy out of me, pushing on me until it feels like I'm a thousand feet down at the bottom of a cold dark ocean. As a kid, I thought this was normal; I thought everybody had times when they barely had the energy to talk, when they stayed quiet for days. When I got older, I discovered the darkness had a name: clinical depression. It's genetic, and our family curse: my maternal grandmother committed suicide; my mom suffers from it as well. Today, I control it with the help of medication; back then, I had Mom. When the dark wave overtook me, she would be there, letting me know she knew how I felt. It wasn't anything big; maybe she'd make me a bowl of chicken-noodle soup, or take me for a walk, or just let me climb up on her lap. But it helped a lot. Those moments bonded us, and fueled within me an endless desire to make her proud, to show her what I could do. To this day, when I reflect on the deepest reasons I wanted to be an athlete, I think a lot of it came from a powerful desire to make her proud. *Look, Ma!*

When I was eleven or so, I made an important dis-covery. It happened while I was skiing at Wildcat

Mountain, New Hampshire, where we went every winter weekend. Wildcat is a famously brutal place to ski: steep, icy, with some of the worst weather on the continent. It's located in the White Mountains, directly across the valley from Mount Washington, where the highest winds in North America are regularly recorded. This day was typical: horrendous winds, stinging sleet, freezing rain. I was skiing with the rest of the Wildcat ski team, riding up the chairlift and skiing down a bamboo-pole racecourse, over and over. Until for some reason I got a strange idea, almost a compulsion.

Don't take the chairlift. Walk up instead.

So I got out of the chairlift line and started walking. It wasn't easy. I had to carry my skis on my shoulder, and chip steps in the ice with the toe of my heavy ski boots. My teammates, riding up in the lift, looked down at me as if I'd gone insane, and in a way they were right: a scrawny eleven-year-old was racing against the chairlift. Some of my teammates joined me. We were John Henry against the steam engine; our legs against the horsepower of that big spinning motor. And so we raced: up, up, up, one step at a time. I remember feeling the pain burning in my legs, feeling my heart in my throat, and also feeling something more profound: I realized that I could keep going. I didn't have to stop. I could hear the pain, but I didn't have to listen to it.

That day awakened something in me. I discovered when I went all out, when I put 100 percent of my energy into some intense, impossible task—when my heart was jackhammering, when lactic acid was sizzling through my muscles—that's when I felt good, normal, balanced. I'm sure a scientist would explain it by saying the endorphins and adrenaline temporarily altered my brain chemistry, and maybe they'd be right. All I knew, though, was the more I pushed myself, the better I felt. Exertion was my escape. I think that's why I was always able to keep up with guys who were bigger and stronger, and who scored better on physiological tests. Because tests can't measure willingness to suffer.

Let me sum up my early sporting career. First I was a skier—regionally, nationally ranked, Olympic hopeful. I raced bikes in the off-season to keep in shape, and I won some age-group races in high school—I was a solid bike racer, but certainly not national-level. Then, during my sophomore year at the University of Colorado, I broke my back while dry-land training with the ski team, ending my ski career. While I was recovering, I funneled all my energy into the bike, and made Big Discovery Number Two: I *loved* bike racing. Bike racing combined the thrill of skiing with the savvy of chess. Best of all (for me), it rewarded the ability to suffer. The more you could suffer, the better you did. One year later, I was 1993 national collegiate cycling champion. By the following summer, I was one of the better amateur riders in the country, a member of the U.S. National Team, and an Olympic hopeful. It was crazy, unlikely, and it felt like I'd found my destiny.

By the spring of 1994, life was beautifully simple. I was twenty-three years old, living in a small apartment in Boulder, subsisting on ramen noodles and Boboli ready-made pizza crusts covered with peanut butter. The national team paid only a small stipend, so to make ends meet I started a business called Flatiron Hauling, the assets of which consisted of myself and a 1973 Ford flatbed truck. I placed an ad in the *Boulder Daily Camera* with the slogan that might've been my athletic motto: "No Job Too Small or Tough." I hauled stumps, scrap metal, and, once, what looked to be a metric ton of dog shit out of someone's backyard. Even so, I felt fortunate to be where I was: standing at the bottom of bike racing's huge staircase, looking up, wondering how high I might climb.

That's when I met Lance. It was May 1994, a rainy afternoon in Wilmington, Delaware, and I was entered in a bike race called the Tour DuPont: 12 days, 1,000 miles, 112 riders, including five of the top nine teams in the world. Lance and I were roughly the same age, but we wanted different things. Lance was out to win. I wanted to see if I could keep up, if I belonged with the big kids.

He was a big deal already. He'd won the world championship one-day race the previous fall in Oslo, Norway. I'd kept the *VeloNews* with his picture and I knew his story by heart: the fatherless Texan born to a teenage mom, the triathlon prodigy who'd switched to bike racing. The articles all used the words "brazen" and "brash" to describe his personality. I'd seen how Armstrong celebrated at the finish line in Oslo with a touchdown dance: blowing kisses, punching the air, showboating for the crowd. Some people—okay, pretty much all people—thought Lance was cocky. But I liked his energy, his in-your-face style. When people asked Armstrong if he was the second Greg LeMond, he would say, "Nope, I'm the first Lance Armstrong."

There were lots of Lance stories being traded around.

One involved the time when world champion Moreno Argentin accidentally called Armstrong by the wrong name, mistaking him for Lance's teammate Andy Bishop. Armstrong blew a gasket. "Fuck you, Chiappucci!" he yelled, calling Argentin by the name of his teammate. Another took place in the previous year's Tour DuPont. A Spanish rider tried to nudge American Scott Mercier off the road, and Armstrong had come to his countryman's defense, racing up to the Spanish guy and telling him to back off—and the Spanish guy actually did. All the stories were really the same story: Lance being Lance, the headstrong American cowboy storming the castle walls of European cycling. I loved hearing these stories, because I was dreaming of storming those castle walls, too.

The day before the race started, I walked around staring at faces I'd only seen in cycling magazines. The Russian Olympic gold medalist Viatcheslav Ekimov, with his rock-star mullet and his Soviet scowl. Mexican climber Raúl Alcalá, the silent assassin who'd won the previous year's race. George Hincapie, a lanky, sleepy-eyed New Yorker who'd been tipped as the next big American racer. There was even three-time Tour de France champion Greg LeMond, in his final year before retirement but still looking bright-eyed and youthful.

You can tell a rider's fitness by the shape of his ass and the veins in his legs, and these asses were bionic, smaller and more powerful than any I'd ever seen. Their leg veins looked like highway maps. Their arms were toothpicks. On their bikes, they could slither through the tightest pack of riders at full speed, one hand on the handlebars. Looking at them was inspiring; they were like racehorses.

Looking at myself—that was a different feeling. If they were thoroughbreds, I was a work pony. My ass was big; my legs showed zero veins. I had narrow shoulders, ski-racer thighs, and thick arms that fit into my jersey sleeves like sausages into casing. Plus, I pedaled with a potato-masher stroke, and because I was on the small side, I had a tendency to tilt my head slightly back to see over other riders, which people said gave me a slightly surprised look, as if I wasn't quite sure where I was. The plain truth was, I had no real business being in the Tour DuPont. I didn't have the power, experience, or the bike-handling skills to compete with the European pros, much less beat them over twelve days.

But I did have one shot: the prologue time trial—each rider racing alone, against the clock. It was a short stage, only 2.98 miles long, a hilly course with several wicked sections of cobbles, and turns tight enough to require the hay-bale crash padding you usually see in a ski race. While short, the prologue was viewed as an important yardstick of ability, since each rider would be revving his engine to the max. The day before the race, I rode the course a half-dozen times. I examined each curve, memorizing the entry and exit angles, closing my eyes, visualizing myself in the race.

The morning of the prologue, it started raining. I stood near the start ramp, chatting with my U.S. national team coach, a smiley thirty-two-year-old named Chris Carmichael. Carmichael was a nice guy, but he was more of a cheerleader than a coach. He liked to repeat certain pet phrases over and over, like they were lyrics to a pop song. Before the prologue, Chris serenaded me with his entire greatest-hits album: *Ride hard, stay within yourself, don't forget to breathe*. I wasn't really listening to him, though. I was thinking about the rain, and how it was going to make the cobbles as slick as ice, and how most of my competitors would be afraid to go hard through the corners. I was thinking, I might be a rookie, but I have two advantages: I know how to ski race, and I've got nothing to lose.

I launched off the ramp and cut into the first corner at full speed, with Carmichael following in a team car. I kept pushing, going right to the limit and staying there. I can tell I'm at the limit when I can taste a little bit of blood in my mouth, and that's how I stayed, right on the edge. This moment is why I fell in love with bike racing, and why I still love it—the mysterious surprises that can happen when you give everything you've got. You push yourself to the absolute limit—when your muscles are screaming, when your heart is going to explode, when you can feel the lactic acid seeping into your face and hands—and then you nudge yourself a little bit further, and then a little further still, and then, things happen. Sometimes you blow up; other times you hit that limit and can't get past it. But sometimes you get past it, and you get into a place where the pain increases so much that you disappear completely. I know that sounds kind of zen but that's what it feels like. Chris used to tell me to stay within myself, but I never understood the sense of that. To me the whole point is to go *out* of yourself, to push over and over until you arrive somewhere new, somewhere you could barely imagine before.

I accelerated into the corners like a race car, skidding

on the cobbles but somehow staying upright and out of the hay bales. I dug frantically on the hills; tucked and drove on the flats. I could feel the lactic acid building up, moving through my body, filling up my legs, my arms, my hands, under my fingernails—good, fresh pain. There was one last 90-degree turn, from cobbles onto pavement. I made it, straightened and gunned it for the line. As I crossed, I glanced at the clock: 6 minutes, 32 seconds.

Third place.

I blinked. Looked again.

Third place.

Not 103rd. Not 30th. Third place.

Carmichael was stunned, shell-shocked. He hugged me, saying, "You are one crazy motherfucker." Then we stood and watched the rest of the riders, assuming that my time would gradually be eclipsed many times over. But as rider after rider crossed the line, my time stayed up.

Ekimov—three seconds behind me.

Hincapie—three seconds behind me.

LeMond—one second ahead of me.

Armstrong—eleven seconds behind me.

When the final rider finished, I was in sixth place.

The following day, as the peloton rolled out of Wilmington for stage 1, I wondered if some of the pros would talk to me; perhaps they'd say hello, offer a friendly word. Not one of them did—not Alcalá, not Ekimov, not LeMond. I was disappointed, and also relieved. I didn't mind being anonymous. I reminded myself that I was just an amateur, a work pony, a nobody.

Then, about ten miles into the race, I felt a friendly tap on my back. I turned, and there was Lance's face, two feet from mine. He looked straight into my eyes.

"Hey Tyler, good ride yesterday."

I'm far from the first person to point this out, but Lance has a compelling way of talking. First he likes to pause for about half a second right before he says something. He just looks at you, checking you, and also letting you check him.

"Thanks," I said.

He nodded. Something passed between us—respect? Recognition? Whatever it was, it felt pretty cool. For the first time, I got a feeling that I might belong.

We kept riding. Being a newbie in a pro peloton is a bit like being a student driver on a Los Angeles freeway: move fast, or else. Halfway through the stage, inevitably, I messed up. I moved to the side, and accidentally cut off a big European guy, nearly hitting his front wheel, and he got pissed off. Not just angry, but theatrically angry, waving his arms and screaming at me in a language I didn't understand. I turned to try to apologize, but that made me swerve even more and now European Guy was screaming louder, riders were starting to stare, and I was dying of embarrassment. European Guy rode up next to me, so he could yell directly in my face.

Then someone moved between the angry European and me. Lance. He put his hand on European Guy's shoulder and gave a gentle but firm push, sending a clear message—*back off*—and as he did, he stared European Guy down, daring him to do something about it. I was so grateful to Lance I could have hugged him.

As the race went on over the next few days, I slid back with the other work ponies. Lance got stronger. He ducked a potential disaster at the end of the stage 5 time trial when, because of a screwup with traffic control, he was nearly crushed by a dump truck that was driving onto the racecourse. But Lance saw the truck coming, and managed to slip through an opening with an inch to spare on either side. He finished second that day to Ekimov. Afterward the press wanted to talk about the near miss— he'd almost died! But not Lance. Instead, he talked about how he should've won the race. That was Lance in a nutshell: cheat death, then get pissed you didn't win.

All in all, I was pretty impressed with the Texan. But what really impressed me happened that July. That's when, from the safe distance of a TV screen, I watched Lance ride the Tour de France—the toughest race on earth, three weeks, 2,500 miles. For the first few days, he did pretty well. Then came stage 9, a 64-kilometer time trial: the race of truth, each rider sent off at one-minute intervals, alone against the clock. I watched in disbelief as Lance got passed by Tour champion Miguel Indurain. Actually "got passed" doesn't do justice to how much faster the Spaniard was going. It was closer to "got blown into a ditch." In the space of thirty seconds, Indurain went from being twenty bike lengths behind Lance to being so far ahead that he'd almost ridden out of camera frame. Lance lost more than six minutes that day, a massive amount. A few days later he abandoned—the second year in a row he'd failed to finish.

I watched, thinking, *Holy shit*. I knew how strong Lance had been only two months before, and how well he could suffer. I'd seen him do things on a bike I could barely imagine, and yet here came Indurain, making Lance look like a work pony.

I had always heard the Tour de France was hard, but that's when I realized that it required an unimaginable level of strength, toughness, and suffering. That was also the moment when I realized that, more than anything, I wanted to ride it.

I'd hoped my little success at the Tour DuPont might catch the eye of a professional team. It seemed I was wrong. I spent the summer of 1994 continuing to ride as an amateur, listening to Coach Carmichael's increasingly bland cheerleading. Off the bike, I ran the hauling business, painted houses, and waited for my phone to ring.

One afternoon in October, while I was painting my neighbor's house, my phone rang. I sprinted inside, still splattered with paint, and picked up the receiver with my fingertips. The voice on the other end was gravelly, commanding, and impatient—the voice of God, if God had woken up on the wrong side of the bed.

"So what's it gonna take to get you on our team?" Thomas Weisel said.

I tried to play cool. I had never talked to him before, but like everybody I knew Weisel's story: fifty-something Harvard-trained millionaire investment banker, former national-level speed skater, masters bike racer, and, above all else, a winner. In the coming decade these guys would be a dime a dozen, enduro jock CEOs who traded golf clubs for a racing bike. But Weisel was the original of the species. For him, life was a race, and it was won by the toughest, the strongest, the guy who could do what it takes. Weisel's motto was *Get it fucking done*. I can still hear that gravelly voice: *Just go get it done. Get it fucking done.*

What Weisel wanted to do was build an American team to win the Tour de France. As more than one person had pointed out, it was the equivalent of starting a French baseball team and attempting to win the World Series. Plus, you couldn't just start a team and enter the Tour— your team had to be invited by the organizers, an invitation based on getting results in big European races. This was not easy. In fact, it was so difficult that Weisel's main sponsor, Subaru, had abandoned him the previous fall, leaving Weisel alone, just him against the world. In other words, exactly where he liked to be.

Here's a story about Weisel: When he was in his late forties, he decided to get serious about cycling. So he hired Eddie Borysewicz, the Olympic team's cycling coach and the godfather of American bike racing.* Twice

---

* Borysewicz was best known for importing Eastern European training methods to the United States—including some that were more than a little questionable. Prior to the 1984 Olympic Games, Borysewicz arranged blood transfusions for the U.S. Olympic cycling team in a Ramada Inn in Carson, California. The team went on to win nine medals, including four golds. While transfusions were not technically against the rules at the time, the United States Olympic Committee condemned the procedure, calling the transfusions "unacceptable, unethical, and illegal as far as the USOC is concerned."

The scandal and ensuing publicity seem to have scared Borysewicz straight: Hamilton and teammate Andy Hampsten agree that the team was clean during Eddie B's 1995–96 tenure as director, and that he frequently warned them against "getting involved with that shit."

a week, Weisel flew from San Francisco to San Diego to train with Eddie B from 10 a.m. until 5 p.m. During the winter, Weisel kept a photo of his main rival pinned up on his weight room wall "to remind me why I was working so hard." Weisel went on to win three age-group masters world championships and five national titles on the road and the track.

"Was it worth it?" a friend asked afterward.

"Yeah, but only because I won," Weisel said.

Weisel's personality was similar to Lance's (later, on Postal, we riders would frequently confuse one's voice for the other's). In fact, back in 1990, Weisel had hired Lance for his pro-am cycling team, called Subaru-Montgomery, when Lance was just nineteen. The two hadn't gotten along; most attributed it to the fact that they were too much alike. Weisel had let Armstrong go; Armstrong had become world champion three years later—a rare example of Weisel letting his emotions get ahead of a business opportunity.

Weisel told me how he'd signed other good American riders—Darren Baker, Marty Jemison, and Nate Reiss—and hired Eddie B to coach. The team would be called Montgomery-Bell. How much did I want for one year? I hesitated. If I went too high, I might lose this. But I didn't want to go cheap, either. So I named a figure in the middle. Thirty thousand dollars.

"You got it," Weisel growled, and I thanked him profusely and hung up the phone. I called my parents to tell them the news: I was officially a professional bike racer.

Year one of the Weisel Experiment went pretty well. We spent 1995 racing mostly in the States, with a couple of trips to Europe to enter smaller races. The team was a mix: mostly younger Americans, with a sprinkling of middling European racers. Though Eddie B tended to be disorganized at times (we got lost a lot traveling to and from races; the race schedule kept changing), the craziness made it fun, helped the team become tighter, and besides, most of us didn't know any different. One afternoon, a soigneur (team assistant) gave me my first injection. It was perfectly legal—iron and vitamin B—but it was also a little unnerving, the sight of a needle going into my ass. He told me it was for my health, because I was depleted from all the racing I'd been doing. After all, bike racing was the hardest sport on earth; it put you out of balance; the vitamins would help restore what was lost. Like with astronauts, he said.

Besides, we riders had far more important things to worry about. We competed to see who could do the best impression of Eddie B's Polish accent, where "you" was a Brooklynese "youse" and every verb was plural. *Youse must attacks now! Youse must attacks now!* Weisel was a constant presence at the bigger races, almost another coach. When we won, he would get teary-eyed, and hug everyone as if we'd just won the Tour de France. I probably made him cry when we traveled to a small race in Holland, a contest called the Teleflex Tour, and I managed to win the overall. Not the biggest race in the world, but it felt good—another sign that I might belong in this sport. Besides, I needed the money: I had my eye on a house in Nederland, Colorado, a small, sleepy town just outside Boulder. The house wasn't anything fancy, just fifteen hundred square feet, with a small porch where I could see the mountains. But to me it meant a sense of permanence, a place to call my own.

In early 1996 Weisel hired former Olympic gold medalist Mark Gorski as general manager. Within a few months Gorski delivered the big news: the U.S. Postal Service had agreed to a three-year contract to be the team's title sponsor, with budget increases built in so the team could grow. Weisel and Gorski got busy stocking the roster with more young riders, capping it with Andy Hampsten, who was the most accomplished American cyclist this side of Greg LeMond. Hampsten had won the Tour of Italy, the Tour of Switzerland, and the Tour of Romandie.

The plan for 1996–97 was to establish Postal's European credentials. We'd enter more big races, and hopefully, by 1997, earn an invitation to what Weisel liked to call the Tour de Fucking France. We fed off Weisel's determination. We felt optimistic and energized, especially with Hampsten leading us. That spring of '96 we headed to Europe feeling optimistic. We knew it'd be tough, but we'd find a way to get it done.

We had no idea.

Chapter 2

REALITY

AT FIRST, WE TOLD ourselves it was jet lag. Then the weather. Then our diet. Our horoscopes. Anything to avoid facing the truth about Postal's performance in the bigger European races in 1996: we were getting crushed.

It wasn't that we were losing; it was the way we were losing. You can grade your performance in a race the same way you would grade a test in school. If you cross the finish line in the lead group, then you earned an A: you might not have won, but you never got left behind. If you are in the second group, you get a B—not great, but far from terrible; you only got left behind once. If you're in the third group, you get a C, and so on. Each race is really a bunch of smaller races, contests that always have one of two results: you either keep up, or you don't.

As a team, Postal was scoring D's and F's. We did fairly well in America, but our performance in the big European races seemed to follow the same pattern: the race would start, and the speed would crank up, and up, and up.

Pretty soon we were hanging on for dear life. Pack-fill, we called ourselves, because our only function was to make the back group of the peloton bigger. We had no chance to win, no chance to attack or affect the race in a meaningful way; we were just grateful to survive. The reason was that the other riders were unbelievably strong. They defied the rules of physics and bike racing. They did things I'd never seen, or even imagined seeing.

For instance, they could attack, alone, and hold off a charging peloton for hours. They could climb at dazzling speed, even the bigger guys who didn't look like climbers. They could perform at their absolute best day after day, avoiding the usual peaks and valleys. They were circus strongmen.

For me, the guy who stood out was Bjarne Riis, a six-foot-tall, 152-pound Dane nicknamed the Eagle. Riis had a big bald head, and intense blue eyes that rarely blinked. He spoke seldom, and usually cryptically. His focus was so intense that it sometimes looked as if he were in a trance. But the strangest thing about Riis, by far, was the arc of his career.

For most of his career, Riis was a decent racer: solid, but rarely a contender in the big races. Then, in 1993, at twenty-seven, he went from average to incredible. He finished fifth in the 1993 Tour, with a stage win; in 1995, he finished third. By 1996, some observers believed he might even be able to defeat the sport's reigning king, five-time defending champion Miguel Indurain.

I remember one of the first times I saw him up close, in the spring of 1997. We were going hard up some brutally steep climb, and Riis was working his way through the group, except he was pushing a gigantic gear. The rest of us were spinning along at the usual rhythm of around 90 rpms, and here comes Bjarne, blank-faced, churning away at 40 rpms, pushing a gear that I couldn't imagine pushing. Then I realized: he's training. The rest of us are going full bore, either trying to win or trying to hang on, and he's *training*. As Riis went by, I couldn't resist. I said, "Hey, how's it going?" to see if he'd react. He gave me a glare and just kept riding.

You looked at Riis, you looked at the dozens of Riis look-alikes that made up the peloton, and you couldn't help but wonder what was going on. I mean, I was green, but I wasn't an idiot. I knew some bike racers doped. I'd read about it—albeit limitedly, in this pre-Internet age—in the pages of *VeloNews*. I'd heard about steroids (which mystified me at the time, since bike racers don't have big muscles); I'd heard about riders popping amphetamines, about syringes tucked in jersey pockets. And lately I'd heard about erythropoietin, EPO, the blood booster that added, some said, 20 percent to endurance by causing the body to produce more oxygen-carrying red blood cells.*

---

* Historical note: Doping and cycling have been intertwined since the sport's earliest days. In the first part of the twentieth century, cyclists used stimulants that affected the brain (cocaine, ether, amphetamines), reducing feelings of fatigue. In the 1970s, new drugs like steroids and corticoids focused on the body's muscles and connective tissues, adding strength and reducing recovery time. But the real doping breakthrough happened when the focus shifted to the blood—specifically to increasing its oxygen-carrying capacity.

Erythropoietin, or EPO, is a naturally occurring hormone that stimulates the bone marrow to produce more oxygen-carrying red blood cells. Commercially developed in the mid-eighties to help dialysis and cancer patients who suffered from anemia, it was quickly adopted by athletes—and for good

The rumors didn't impress me as much as the speed—the relentless, brutal, mechanical speed. I wasn't alone. Andy Hampsten was achieving the same power outputs as previous years, years when he'd won the big races. Now, producing that same power, he was struggling to stay in the top fifty. Hampsten, who was staunchly anti-doping, and who would soon retire at age thirty-two rather than dope, had a good view of the change.

ANDY HAMPSTEN: In the mid-eighties, when I came up, riders were doping but it was still possible to compete with them. It was either amphetamines or anabolics—both were powerful, but they had downsides. Amphetamines made riders stupid—they'd launch these crazy attacks, use up all their energy. Anabolics made people bloated, heavy, gave them injuries in the long run, not to mention these horrid skin rashes. They'd be superstrong in the cool weather, in shorter races, but in a long, hot stage race, the anabolics would drag them down. So

reason. A 13-week study of fit recreational cyclists in the *European Journal of Applied Physiology* shows that EPO increased peak power output by 12–15 percent, and increased endurance (time riding at 80 percent of maximum) by 80 percent. Dr. Ross Tucker, who writes for the highly regarded Science of Sport website, estimates that for world-class athletes, EPO improves performance around 5 percent, or roughly the difference between first place in the Tour de France and the middle of the pack.

One early risk of EPO was the increased likelihood of funerals. EPO is thought to be behind the deaths of a dozen Dutch and Belgian cyclists in the late eighties and early nineties: their hearts stopped when they could not pump the EPO-thickened blood. Stories from that era tell of riders who set alarm clocks for the middle of the night, so they could wake up and do some pulse-increasing calisthenics.

bottom line, a clean rider could compete in the big three-week tours.

EPO changed everything. Amphetamines and anabolics are nothing compared to EPO. All of a sudden whole teams were ragingly fast; all of a sudden I was struggling to make time limits. By 1994, it was ridiculous. I'd be on climbs, working as hard as I'd ever worked, producing exactly the same power, at the same weight, and right alongside me would be these big-assed guys, and they'd be chatting like we were on the flats! It was completely crazy.*

As the [1996] season went by, there was so much tension at the dinner table—everybody knew what was up, everybody was talking about EPO, everybody could see the writing on the wall. They were looking to me to give them a little guidance. But what could I say?

Nobody sets out wanting to dope. We love our sport because of its purity; it's just you, your bike, the road, the race. And when you enter a world and you begin to sense that doping is going on, your instinctive reaction is to close your eyes, clap your hands over your ears, and work even harder. To rely on the old mystery of bike racing— push to the limit, then push harder, because who knows, today might be better. In fact, I know this sounds strange, but the idea that others doped actually inspired me at first;

* From 1980 to 1990, the average speed of the Tour de France was 37.5 kph; from 1995 to 2005, it increased to an average of 41.6 kilometers per hour. When you account for air resistance, that translates to a 22 percent increase in overall power.

it made me feel noble because I was pure. I would prevail because my cleanness would make me stronger. No job too small or tough.

It was easy to maintain this attitude, because doping simply wasn't discussed—at least, not officially. We'd whisper about it at the dinner table or on rides, but never with our team directors or management or doctors. Every once in a while, an article might appear in a foreign paper and cause a brief commotion, but for the most part everyone pretended that these insane race speeds were normal. It was as if you were staring at someone casually lifting thousand-pound barbells over their heads with one hand, and everybody around you was acting like it was just another day at the office.

Still, we couldn't help but express our worries. There's an oft-told story about how Marty Jemison and I approached Postal doctor Prentice Steffen in 1996 and had a conversation about how fast the races were. Steffen says Marty hinted that the team should start providing some illicit medical enhancements, and that I stood there in support. I have to say, I don't remember this specific incident happening, but I can certainly recall the feeling of being worried, of wondering why the hell these guys were so fast, and wondering what they might be on.[*]

[*] This incident became semi-famous when Steffen recounted it numerous times in the media over the years. Steffen maintains that Jemison was hinting about doping. Jemison says he was frustrated at Steffen's insistence on giving Postal riders no more than aspirin and oral vitamins. "I knew there were legal intravenous vitamins and amino acids, and I put pressure on Steffen to tell me why we weren't doing that," Jemison says. "At that moment, I can honestly say that doping wasn't on my radar. I'd never heard the term 'EPO.' That changed fast, though."

Weisel, as you might imagine, enjoyed losing even less than we did, and his feelings were intensified by the structure of the sport. In baseball or football, the league lends stability to each team. Pro cycling, on the other hand, follows a more Darwinian model: teams are sponsored by big companies, and compete to get into big races. There are no assurances; sponsors can leave, races can refuse to allow teams. The result is a chain of perpetual nervousness: sponsors are nervous because they need results. Team directors are nervous because they need results. And riders are nervous because they need results to get a contract.

Weisel understood this equation. This was his shot for the Tour, and he is not the kind of guy who reacts to losing by patting you on the back and saying, "Don't worry, guys, we'll get 'em tomorrow." No, Weisel was the kind of guy who reacted to losing by getting pissed off. And in 1996 we watched him go from pissed off to white hot to Defcon 5. We started to see him and Eddie B arguing after races. We started to hear the growl.

We better see some good numbers tomorrow, or somebody's gonna be seeing the door.

You guys gotta step it up, starting now!

That was fucking pathetic. What's the problem with you guys?

The nine-day Tour of Switzerland in June was our chance for redemption. We were hopeful; Hampsten, who would co-lead with Darren Baker, had won the race in 1988. Weisel planned to fly over for the big stages to ride in the team car with Eddie B. This was going to be our big opportunity to prove that we belonged.

We got crushed. We hung for a few days, but when the race got serious, we flunked. The telling moment came on stage 4, on the climb of the monstrous Grimsel Pass—26 kilometers long, 1,540 meters gained with a 6 percent grade, ending at the aptly named Lake of the Dead. On the lower slopes, the pack accelerated and we fell away like we had anchors attached to our bikes. Hampsten was the last holdout, hanging tough in a group of twenty, flying up, up the mountain. Weisel and Eddie B yelled encouragement, but it was no use—Hampsten was going full bore, and everybody was simply stronger. The group pulled away, leaving Hampsten behind.

Watching the leaders disappear up the road, Weisel got antsy. Race protocol requires the team car to remain behind the team's leading rider in order to help him with feeding and mechanical problems; violating this rule is unthinkable, the equivalent of a NASCAR pit crew abandoning their post in the middle of a race. But Weisel had no more patience, not for protocol, not for anything. He ordered Eddie B to leave Hampsten, to drive around him, to catch up with the leaders so he could see the fireworks. Weisel wanted to scout new riders for the 1997 team. The engine revved; Hampsten watched in disbelief as the Postal car disappeared up the road. The message was clear: Weisel wasn't going to wait around for losers.

Two days later, at the foot of Susten Pass (17 kilometers at 7.5 percent grade), co-leader Darren Baker blew a tire. I gave him my wheel and by the time I got a replacement, I was alone. I gave everything I had, but couldn't catch up. I spent the day alone, trying to make it under the time limit. I remember seeing desperate riders hanging on to rearview mirrors, hitching rides. I remember telling myself I'd never do that. In the end I missed the cutoff, and the next day I was on a plane back home, wondering if I had what it took.

The Tour of Switzerland was the kind of experience that might have made me think twice about my sport, to wonder why I was working so hard for nothing. I might have been tempted to quit, if bike racing had been the only thing in my life. But it wasn't. You see, a few weeks before that race, I had fallen in love.

Her name was Haven Parchinski; we'd met at the Tour DuPont back in the States that spring; she'd volunteered at the race, checking badges at the hotel dining room. She was beautiful: petite and dark-haired, with a huge smile and hazel eyes that seemed to catch the light. I was nervous about talking with her, so I asked my teammate Marty Jemison's wife, Jill, who worked PR for Postal, to introduce us. It turned out Haven lived in Boston, and worked as an account executive at Hill Holliday, an advertising agency. I started arriving at meals early and having four or five coffees afterward, just to have an excuse to be in the same room. We started to chat, and to flirt. My heart was thumping, and it wasn't the coffee.

The race that year was being dominated by Lance, who'd showed up bigger and stronger than ever.* But in

---

* Armstrong had started working with Italian doctor Michele Ferrari in the fall of 1995. When he showed up for the 1996 season, teammates were surprised at how big he'd become. Armstrong's arms were so big that he had to cut the sleeves of his jersey to fit them; Scott Mercier kidded him about playing for the Cowboys.

one of the last stages of the race, I found myself in the lead group, and I was feeling strong. It's funny how much racing depends on your emotions; my crush on Haven was a shot of rocket fuel. With about four kilometers to go I launched a solo attack and nearly made it to the line before the pack caught me. I won the day's most aggressive rider award, and was called to stand on the podium, and was handed a beautiful bouquet of flowers. That night, I sent the bouquet to Haven's room. At first, she thought it was some kind of mistake. Then she connected the dots, and called to thank me, and we talked for an hour. At the end of the race, there was a party, and afterward I walked her to her room and gave her a goodnight kiss—a single kiss, nothing more, and nothing less—and from that moment on we were together.

We were a good match. Haven wasn't impressed by bike racers, and didn't know a whole lot about cycling, and I loved that. She knew about business, the ad game, politics, the bigger world I'd been missing.

The real test for our new relationship came when Haven went to visit my family in Marblehead for the annual Mountain Goat Invitational Crazy Croquet Tournament in our backyard. Haven dove right in, proved she could take it and dish it out with the best of them. She sent my parents a thank-you note afterward, mentioning that she'd never realized that croquet was a full-contact sport. My folks loved her; they'd often meet her for dinner when I was out of town. We used to joke that with my race schedule, they had more dates with Haven than I did.

Haven's parents were less enthusiastic about our

relationship, maybe because "aspiring bike racer" doesn't look great on a résumé. But they came to a race that July, in Fitchburg, Massachusetts, and I was fortunate enough to win, so they could see that while their daughter might be dating only a bike racer, at least she was dating a decent one. That December I left my little house in Nederland, Colorado, and moved into Haven's place in Boston, though we didn't tell her parents; we pretended I was just visiting.

When I look back, those might have been my happiest days. I was twenty-five years old. I had a budding relationship with Haven, a boisterous new golden retriever pup named Tugboat, and maybe a future racing my bike, if I kept improving. It felt like magic—I pushed the pedals, and this fun, interesting, challenging life was assembling itself around me. Around us.

Over in Europe, there were also hopeful signs that the days of the circus strongmen might be numbered. Riis's 1996 Tour de France victory had been marked by moments of superhuman dominance, and people were whispering about doping. For example, at key moments on big climbs, Riis had done something no one had ever seen: he coasted back to look at the other contenders, almost taunting them, then accelerated away as if on a motorcycle. Around Europe, voices of reason began to speak up. An Italian judicial report had put a spotlight on EPO abuse among pro cyclists in that country; the French newspaper *L'Équipe* had published a series of articles in which riders said they could no longer keep up without taking EPO, which was as yet undetectable in tests. Columnists wrote about how the new drugs were endangering the dignity of the sport. All this pressure fell smack onto the shoulders of Hein Verbruggen, the Dutchman who ran the UCI, cycling's governing body. I hoped the UCI would act, if for no other reason than that I reasoned it might improve my chances of keeping up.

But all that seemed like small potatoes when I heard in early October that Lance had been diagnosed with testicular cancer, which had spread to his abdomen and brain. It was shocking, a reminder of how quickly life can change. The photos of him shook me to the core. I'd just seen him, so big and strong and invincible, winning the Tour DuPont that May. Now he was skinny, bald, scarred. I heard that he had vowed to come back, and my first thought was, *No way*. My second thought was, *Well, if anybody can, it's Lance.*

As the calendar turned toward spring, I found myself looking forward to the 1997 season with new enthusiasm. Weisel was the talk of the cycling world, because he was getting it done. He was signing some of the sport's biggest names. We'd heard he was overhauling the staff and the schedule, and that some of us—hopefully me—would be based full-time in Europe, in a town near the Pyrenees called Girona. As this news arrived, Haven and I talked it over, and tried to figure out how we were going to navigate these changes. One thing we settled on fast: whatever happened, wherever it happened, we'd make it work.

Chapter 3

EURODOGS

I went from thinking one hundred percent that I would never dope to making a decision in ten minutes that I was going to do it.
— *David Millar, former World Champion and Tour de France stage winner*

TO KICK OFF the 1997 season, Thom Weisel gathered the team at his beach house in Oceanside, California, a few miles from where we were holding our training camp. It was Super Bowl Sunday in late January; a perfect blue-sky California day. We stood in his living room, with its picture windows and its million-dollar ocean views. But I paid zero attention to that, because the view inside was more impressive.

There was Olympic gold medalist Viatcheslav Ekimov, his blond mullet in midseason form. There was Jean-Cyril Robin, newly signed from the powerful French Festina team, looking every inch the Tour contender. There was

Adriano Baffi, a muscled strongman from the Mapei team. Eddie B had been demoted to assistant director, replaced by a friendly Dane named Johnny Weltz. Hampsten was gone, having retired. Team doctor Prentice Steffen was gone too, replaced by Dr. Pedro Celaya, a dapper Spaniard with a warm manner and soft brown eyes.*

Just like that, the original Postal team became Postal 2.0: a gleaming, state-of-the-art European model. Looking around, I felt two emotions. The first was a thrill; with these guys on our team, we had a genuine shot at making it into the Tour de France. The second was nervousness: Did I belong with guys of this caliber? Did I have what it took to be a good support rider—what was called a *domestique*, or servant? Could I maybe even make the Tour team, if we made it that far?

At some point, Weisel poured a glass of red wine and raised it. We went quiet, and listened as he made one of his blunt, growling *go get it fucking done* speeches. The football game was on TV, and Weisel made the connection—the Tour de France was our Super Bowl, and we were going to get there, no matter what.

Weisel and Weltz laid out the plan: training would be harder, more organized, more purposeful. I and four

---

* After he was let go, Steffen protested via a letter sent to Postal team manager Mark Gorski that read, in part, "What could a Spanish doctor, completely unknown to the organization, offer that I can't or won't? Doping is the fairly obvious answer." Postal responded via its lawyers, informing Steffen that he would be sued if he made any public statements that caused financial damage to the Postal team. Steffen consulted a lawyer and decided to drop the matter.

other Americans—Scott Mercier, Darren Baker, Marty Jemison, and George Hincapie—would move to Girona. Our racing schedule would be more ambitious; we'd target the prestigious classic Liège–Bastogne–Liège, return to the Tour of Switzerland, and, if we did well enough, ride in our first Tour de France in July. Weisel's goal was clear: we would prove that Postal belonged in Europe. We wouldn't knock on the door anymore; we would kick the bastard off its hinges.

At some point in the party, I spotted a plate of chocolate chip cookies. I was conscious of my weight like any rider, but we had been training hard, and these were awfully good-looking cookies—crispy on the edges, a little underdone in the middle, just the way I like them. I couldn't resist. I reached for one, munched it slowly— perfection. Then I took another. As I chewed, I got a strange feeling I was being watched. I looked up to see the new team doctor, Pedro Celaya, watching me closely from across the room, measuring the moment as surely as if he were taking my temperature. Pedro smiled at me, and slowly waggled a finger in a humorous but firm way: No no! I smiled back, pretending to hide the cookie under my shirt, and he laughed.

I liked Pedro immediately. Unlike Steffen, whom I'd found distant and touchy, Pedro was like your favorite uncle. He looked you in the eyes; he asked how you felt; he remembered little things. He was a slight, pleasant-looking man with an unruly, graying thatch of hair and a playful grin. To him, life seemed a great entertainment; he was always ready for a laugh. His English might have been imperfect, but he was a brilliant conversationalist because he seemed to sense what I was feeling before I felt it.

One of our first serious conversations had to do with my blood. Pedro explained that hematocrit was the percentage of blood that contains red blood cells. He explained a new UCI rule that required any rider whose hematocrit exceeded 50 percent—a probable sign of EPO use—to sit out fifteen days. Because there was as yet no EPO test, exceeding 50 percent was not considered doping; instead, UCI president Hein Verbruggen called it a health issue, terming the suspension "a hematocrit holiday."*

So Pedro asked me if he could please draw a small amount of blood, to check my hematocrit. He did, transferred the blood into a few narrow glass tubes, and inserted the tubes into a device the size of a toaster—a centrifuge. I heard a whirring sound; Pedro extracted the tubes and examined the hatchmark on the side.

"Not too bad," he said. "You are 43."

I remember being struck by Pedro's wording: it wasn't "You scored a 43" or "Your level is 43," it was "*You are 43.*" Like I was a stock, and 43 was my price. Only later would I find out how accurate this really was.

But to be honest, I wasn't paying a lot of attention

---

* Verbruggen, a former sales manager for Mars candy bars, likened the new rule to blood-testing paint-factory workers for lead exposure, just to make sure nobody got sick. When others pointed out that Verbruggen was essentially legalizing doping with EPO (as one Italian team director put it, the new rule was the equivalent of allowing everyone to go into a bank and steal as long as they kept it under $1,000), Verbruggen, who was famous for his short temper, called the analysis "bullshit" and told them to "shut up." Verbruggen has repeatedly and strenuously denied this allegation and sued former WADA president Dick Pound in 2009 when he questioned UCI's efforts to combat doping. The case was settled out of court.

at the time. I was more concerned with immediate things; the upcoming European season, planning, packing, training, seeing where I fit into the newly outfitted team. Scott Mercier was one of the older guys on the team, a former Olympian, and more savvy than I was at the time. I'll let him describe his encounter with our new doctor.

SCOTT MERCIER: I'd never had a doctor ask me for blood before, so I wasn't sure what to expect. But I knew that the only way to raise hematocrit was to take EPO, or get a transfusion. So [Celaya] takes me to his hotel room and we do the test. When he looks at my number, he starts shaking his head.

"Oooooh la la!" Pedro says. "You are 39. To be professional in Europe, you need to be 49, maybe 49.5."

I understood what that meant; he had to be talking about EPO. But I decided to play dumb, to see what the doctor would say.

"How will I do that?" I ask, and Pedro smiles.

"Specialty vitamins," he says. "Why don't we talk about it later?"

When we got to Europe, I had my eyes open. I knew about EPO, I knew it had to be refrigerated. Sure enough, there's a refrigerator in the team mechanic's truck. It's got some drinks, some ice, and, on the lower shelf, a black plastic box, like a tackle box, with a padlock. If you picked it up and shook it, you could hear the vials pinging together. I started calling it "the specialty vitamin lunchbox."

Anybody could see the decision that had been

made at the top, and where the team was headed. It was clear as day. Even so, you don't really want to believe it; you ignore it and try to keep within yourself. For a while. Later that spring, in May, I had a four-week break between races. Pedro came to my hotel room one night and handed me a Ziploc filled with about thirty pills along with some clear liquid in glass vials. He told me they were steroids. "They make you strong, like a bull," he said. "Strong like never before."

I thought about it a long time. A tough decision, and in the end I didn't take the pills and I quit at the end of the year. My heart wasn't in it. What made the difference for me is that I was already twenty-eight; I'd had a good career; I had some options for going forward in my life. I went into business, have done pretty well. Even so, I've wrestled with that decision for fourteen years. I don't blame people who did it in the least—I get why they did it. I mean, look at Tyler—look at how well he did in that world! It's been strange watching that from afar, wondering what might have been, if I'd made a different choice.

In February 1997, a couple of weeks after training camp ended, I headed across the Atlantic. I remember looking out the window of the plane and seeing Spain spread out beneath me, and feeling my stomach lurch. I was nervous. I was about to ride in three races in the south of Spain; then I would meet up with Haven in Barcelona and we'd drive to the new apartment in Girona we were going to share with the other Postal riders. I was nervous about living in Europe, about my still-new relationship with Haven, and about my nonexistent Spanish language skills. But mostly I was nervous about the fact that there were twenty riders on Postal and room for just nine on the Tour team. I wanted to be one of them.

I landed and dove straight into the fire: the five-day Ruta del Sol, the one-day Luis Puig race, then the five-day Tour of Valencia. It was brutal: windy, hot, unbelievably fast, rolling across the Spanish scrublands and coast, the brown and blue scenery. That was when I saw the white bags for the first time. They showed up at the end of each race, brought out by the soigneurs, who kept them in the fridge in the mechanic's truck. They were small, the size of a lunch bag a kid might take to school, folded neatly at the top. The soigneurs didn't make a big deal out of them— that, in a way, was what made it seem big, because they were so matter-of-fact, so routine. They were handed to certain riders as they left the team to go home.

Some riders got them. Some didn't.

The first time I noticed the white bags, it got my attention. After two races, I started looking for them. They were given only to the more veteran riders on the team. The guys I thought of as the A team. That's when I felt a sinking realization: I was on the B team.

It was around this time that I started hearing the phrase "riding paniagua" (pronounced PAN=ee=ah=gwa). Sometimes it was delivered in a slightly depressed tone, as if the speaker were talking about riding a particularly slow and stubborn donkey. *I might've finished higher, but I was riding paniagua*. Other times, it was mentioned as a point of pride. *I finished in the first group of thirty and I was paniagua*. I came to discover that it was really *pan y agua*—"bread and water." From that, I made the obvious conclusion: riding without chemical assistance in the pro peloton was so rare that it was worth pointing out.

I tried to ignore the white bags at first, but I quickly came to hate them. I thought about them often. When I felt an A-team rider pass me, I thought of the white bags. When I felt exhausted and ready to drop, I thought of the white bags. When I worked my ass off and still couldn't come close to competing in the race, I thought of the white bags. In a way they served as my fuel; they made me push myself harder than I've ever pushed, because I wanted to prove that I was better, I was stronger than some little bag. I went to the edge, tasted the blood in my mouth, day after day. And for a while, it worked.

Then I started to break down.

Here's an interesting number: one thousand days. It's roughly the number of days between the day I became professional and the day I doped for the first time. Talking to other riders of this era and reading their stories, it seems to be a pattern: those of us who doped mostly started during our third year. First year, neo-pro, excited to be there, young pup, hopeful. Second year, realization. Third year, clarity—the fork in the road. Yes or no. In or out. Everybody has their thousand days; everybody has their choice.

In some ways, it's depressing. But in other ways, I think it's human. One thousand mornings of waking up with hope; a thousand afternoons of being crushed. A thousand days of paniagua, bumping painfully against the wall at the edge of your limits, trying to find a way past. A thousand days of getting signals that doping is okay, signals from powerful people you trust and admire, signals that say *It'll be fine* and *Everybody's doing it*. And beneath all that, the fear that if you don't find some way to ride faster, then your career is over. Willpower might be strong, but it's not infinite. And once you cross the line, there's no going back.

I raced Ruta del Sol paniagua. I was determined to prove my worth—maybe too eager. The sun was hot, the pace was blazing. For five days I went to my limits and hung there, trying to keep up with the strongmen. I felt my body begin to weaken, and I pushed harder. I dug deep, found a second wind. Then a third. Then a fourth.

Then there were no more winds left. The peloton seemed like it was made up of a hundred Bjarne Riises, a freight train. I felt myself losing strength, drying up like a leaf. I had been in Europe for all of two weeks, and the writing was on the wall. I was starting to feel desperate. I'd always risen to the challenge; I'd always been able to gut it out. *No job too small or tough*. And now, I wasn't tough enough.

At this point I could tell you all about what an honest person I am. I could tell stories about when I was kid, growing up on High Street in Marblehead, how we always played fair, no matter what the game. I could tell you about the honor of my grandfather, who served in the U.S. Navy, or I could tell you about the time I got caught breaking the rules by reselling ski-lift tickets in high school, and had to write forty letters of apology and do volunteer work, and how I learned my lesson and swore to always be a good person, and how I've tried my best to keep that vow.

But that wouldn't be honest, because in my opinion this decision isn't really about honor or character. I know wonderful people who doped; I know questionable people who decided not to. For me, the only fact that mattered was that for a thousand days I had been cheated out of my livelihood, and there was no sign that things were going to get better. So I did what many others had done before me. I joined the brotherhood.

Actually, they came to me. Just after the Ruta del Sol, Pedro came to visit me in my hotel room. My roommate, Peter Meinert Nielsen, was at dinner, so we could talk in private. Pedro was wearing what he usually wore at races: a vest with lots of pockets, like a fly fisherman might use. He sat down and asked me the question he always asked: *How are you, Tyler?* He was always so good at asking that question; he made you feel how much he cared. So I told him the truth. I was wiped out. I could barely make it to the shower. I didn't have anything left.

Pedro didn't say anything at first. He just looked at me—or, to be more accurate, looked into me with those soft, sad brown eyes. Then his hand started rooting around in the fly-fishing vest, and pulled out a brown glass bottle. Slowly, casually, he showed it to me, unscrewed the top, gave an expert tap with his fingertips. A single capsule. A tiny red egg.

"This is not doping," he said. "This is for your health. To help you recover."

I nodded. He was still holding the capsule. I could see it was filled with liquid.

"If you were racing tomorrow, I would not give you this. But it is totally okay if you take it now and race the day after tomorrow," he said. "It's safe. It will help you recover. Your body needs it."

I understood exactly what Pedro was saying; if I was selected to be drug-tested, I would test positive for the next day. As we both knew, they only tested at races, and the next race didn't start for two days. I put out my hand, and he tipped the capsule into my palm. I waited until he was gone, and then I got a glass of water, and looked at myself in the bathroom mirror.

This is not doping. This is for your health.

The race, the Luis Puig, started two days later with an insanely fast climb, a long, brutal switchback ascent. I fell back, as I'd expected to. But then something happened. As we neared the top of the climb, I noticed I was moving up; I was passing one rider, then three, then ten. Don't get me wrong: I wasn't suddenly superman—I was dying, I was at my absolute limit. But the thing was, the others were dying a little more quickly. When a break formed, I was with the A students.

Objectively, I knew what had happened: the red egg—which I found out later was testosterone—had gone into my bloodstream and kicked off a cascade of beneficial changes: added fluid to my muscles, repaired tiny injuries, created a feeling of well-being. It wasn't just me going up that hill, it was an improved me. A more balanced me. As Pedro would say, a healthier me.

I'm not proud of that decision. I wish with all my heart that I'd been stronger, that I'd dropped that red egg back into the bottle and suffered through another day at the back, paniagua. I wish I'd realized the path I was taking, wish I'd quit the sport, come back to Colorado, finished college, maybe gone to business school, had a different life. But I didn't. I took the pill, and it worked—I rode faster, felt better. I felt good, and not just physically. The red egg was a badge of honor, a sign that Pedro and the team saw my potential. I felt like this was a small step toward making the A team.

I didn't win the race, but I did pretty well. Afterward, I accepted a pat on the back from my director, Johnny Weltz, and then I watched as the white bags were handed out. I watched the A-team riders tuck their white bags into their rollaways, and I felt a sinking sensation.

Apparently, I still had more work to do.

After the Tour of Valencia, we headed to Girona, a walled medieval city of 100,000 people in the foothills of the Pyrenees, and my new home for the next seven months. I picked up Haven at the Barcelona airport and we drove north, eager to see the city, which team director Johnny Weltz had described as a rare jewel. We followed Johnny as he drove the road north from Barcelona. The problem was, Johnny drove like a madman through the mist, accelerating to 100 mph. I did my best to keep up, racing in and out of traffic like a Formula One driver. (Haven later looked back on that ride as a metaphor for our entire European experience: an insane, high-speed chase through the foggy darkness.)

Johnny was right about the city. Our apartment, unfortunately, turned out to be the flaw in the jewel: a dusty set of dormitory-like rooms in a decrepit high-rise.

It would be home for four of us—George Hincapie, Scott Mercier, Darren Baker, and me; Marty Jemison and his wife, Jill, lived a short walk away. We drew straws for rooms; Scott, being the tallest, naturally drew the straw for the smallest room (when he lay in bed, his head and feet could almost touch the opposing walls). The place was filthy, so Haven headed up a cleaning project; we spent our first morning scrubbing and dusting, until the place looked less like a scary dump and more like a college dormitory. We dubbed it, in a tribute to the old *Jeffersons* sitcom, our Dee-Luxe Apartment in the Sky. We called ourselves the Eurodogs.

If our life had been a sitcom, Scott Mercier would have played the Smart One: he was twenty-nine, tall and college-educated, a classy thoroughbred both on and off the bike.

Darren Baker would have been the Edgy One; big, strong, tough as nails, he'd come to the sport after being injured as a runner and proven to be a natural (he'd beaten Lance in a big race back in 1992). Darren was a realist to the bone, a guy who took no BS and who reveled in telling hard truths.

George Hincapie was the Quiet One: a twenty-three-year-old who'd spent the last few years racing at a high level in Europe and who'd been picked as a rising star, specializing in the supertough one-day northern European races known as classics. George didn't say much, but on his bike he was eloquent, combining a liquid pedal stroke with a gritty, never-say-die Belgian mentality. People often mistook George's silence for slowness; as time went by, I found the opposite was true.

He was wiser and more observant than anyone suspected.

That left me as the Scrappy One, the undersized pup who had the most to learn about the sport. The theme of our early days was cluelessness. We had no idea where to train, where to get bikes repaired, where to shop for groceries, how to rent a movie or use an ATM. Thank God, George spoke Spanish, and could patiently guide us through the thornier moments. For the first weeks, whenever we encountered a linguistic obstacle, we would call "George!"—so often that it became a running joke. And George always came through: he was kind and patient.

We quickly became friends, and discovered a truth about our sport: there is no friendship in the world like the friendship of being on a bike-racing team. The reason is one word: *give*. You give all your strength: during the race, you shelter each other, you empty yourself for the sake of another person, and they do the same for you. You give all your time: you travel together, room together, eat every meal together. You ride for hours together every day, knuckle to knuckle. To this day, I can remember how each of my teammates chewed their food, how they fixed their coffee, how they walked when they were tired, how their eyes looked when they were going to have a shitty day or a great day. Other sports teams like to call themselves "families." In bike racing, it's close to true.

Thrown together in this far-away place, the four of us became inseparable. When we traveled to races, we stuck together, causing the rest of the peloton to regard us with the same kind of polite curiosity you might give to four toddlers wandering around your workplace: *Oh look, it's the new Americans—aren't they cute?* Our sense of apartness was increased by the fact that the peloton is essentially one big clique, with a set of detailed rules, most of which we were in the process of breaking.

The rule against air-conditioning, for instance. The Europeans believed A/C to be a dangerous invention that caused illness and dried out the lungs; if someone on the bus or in a hotel room turned on the air-conditioning, it was as if they were giving everyone the bubonic plague.

Or the rule against eating chocolate mousse (causes sweating).

Or the rule against sitting down on a curb (tires out the legs).

Or the rule against passing the salt from hand to hand (it had to be set on the table, lest it bring bad luck).

Or the rule against shaving your legs the night before a big race (your body loses energy regrowing the hair).

George proved to be an ideal roommate for two reasons. First, he was a gadget guy. In an age when portable electronics were still exotic, George was a one-man SkyMall: he owned a portable DVD player, speakers, the latest cell phones, laptops, etc. He was the one who gave me my first cell phone; he taught me how to text.

George also taught me how to be lazy. We didn't call it laziness, of course—we called it "conserving energy," and it was an essential part of being a good bike racer. The rules were simple: stand as little as possible, sleep as much as possible. George was amazing at it, a superman of lounging. Whole days would go by, and he would only be vertical to eat and train. I can still see his long body stretched on the couch, legs up, surrounded by a debris field of his electronic gear. He also saved energy when it came to thinking about food: George ate pizza margherita for lunch and dinner some days; he ate it so often that we began to call him Pizza Margherita. I did my best to copy his energy-conserving habits, but it didn't come naturally: I had more nervous energy to burn off, and besides, I was worried about making the team.

The worries, ironically enough, had started with George, and an overheard conversation. The walls of our *apartamento* were painted cinder block, the floors white Spanish tile. You could not drop a pin without it being heard. If someone whispered, you heard it all over the apartment. And there was some whispering going on, between George and our director, Johnny Weltz.

It was natural that Johnny would visit George: after all, George was one of the team's best riders, our biggest hope for a classics victory that could help propel Postal into the Tour. What was not natural, however, was that Johnny would sometimes show up carrying a white bag. You could hear the paper crinkle. Also, when they spoke privately, they would either whisper or switch to Spanish. While George and Johnny were both fluent in Spanish, this didn't make sense to me—we were all on the same team, why not speak English? I couldn't help but be curious. I saw George put a small foil packet in the back of the fridge, behind the Cokes. One day soon after, when George was out, I couldn't resist. I opened the refrigerator and opened up the foil packet. I saw syringes and ampules labeled EPO.

SCOTT MERCIER: I asked George about it once. He and I were sitting alone in the apartment. All this stuff was happening, and I wanted to know. So I asked him, "Do you have to do the drugs to make it?" He hesitated a long time. George is a quiet guy. He doesn't want conflict. So he felt a little on the spot. But eventually he said, "You gotta figure it out for yourself." And I knew what he meant.

I was figuring it out. In March I roomed with Adriano Baffi at the Tour of Catalunya. This was a big deal for me at the time because Baffi was a veteran, a big name, one of Weisel's hired guns; he'd won five stages at the Tour of Italy, which made him a legend on our team. So I walked into our hotel room and the first sound I heard was a high-pitched *zzzzzzzzz*—the centrifuge. I look in to see Baffi, a handsome, debonair guy, fussing over this small machine exactly like Pedro's, except smaller and nicer— the Brookstone version. Baffi wasn't being secretive about it in the least, just matter-of-fact and precise, like he was fixing an espresso. He peered at the hatch-marks on the side of the tube, and he smiled. "Forty-eight!" he said.

In those situations, I always acted like I knew what they were talking about. I know it sounds weird now— maybe I should've been more honest and asked, *Hey, Adriano, why are you testing your own hematocrit? Doesn't the team doctor do that?* But I wanted to be cool, to fit in. At other races, I'd overhear the A-team riders talking about their hematocrit, comparing numbers, with a lot of oohs and aahs and teasing. They talked about hematocrit all the time, as much as they talked about the weather or the road conditions. The numbers seemed to carry huge meaning: *I'm 43—you don't have to worry about me winning today. But I hear you're a 49—look out!* I would smile and nod, and quickly I figured out just how important hematocrit was. It was not just another number; it was *the* number, capable of making the difference between having a chance at winning and not. This was not particularly good news for me, because my own hematocrit usually tested at a depressing 42. The harder I trained and raced, the lower it dropped.

Still, I didn't do anything. Pedro gave me an occasional red egg at races, but that was it. I would not have dreamed of asking Baffi or another teammate for EPO. It felt like something that was above my station, that had to be earned. So I did what I was good at: I put my head down, gritted my teeth, and kept riding, touching limit and trying to nudge a little past it. I might've been able to ignore what was happening a bit longer if it hadn't been for Marty Jemison.

I knew Marty well and considered him a friend. He was a bit older; he had lived in Europe and raced for a Dutch team before joining Weisel's Montgomery squad in 1995. Marty didn't talk a lot about his previous European experience, but I got the feeling it had been tough being a solo American. Marty was a nice guy; a little touchy at times, perhaps, but on the whole friendly and outgoing (he's since founded a successful bike-travel business). The main thing I knew about Marty, though, is that I could usually beat him. We'd raced against each other many times over the years, and I'd ended up on top maybe 80 percent of the time, especially in time trials, which are considered the best measure of pure strength. There was no disputing it; the gap between our abilities was as stable and reliable as our height.

But in the spring of 1997, the pattern reversed. In training rides, and in early season races, Marty started doing better than me, and it made me nervous. Was he doing something? Did I need to do something too?

In April, I was picked to ride for the team in the year's toughest test yet: Liège–Bastogne–Liège, a cruel 257-kilometer painfest through Belgium's Ardennes region that some consider to be the hardest single-day race on the calendar. I put everything toward preparing for it, figuring it was a golden opportunity to improve my chances of making the Tour team. My goal was to make it into the first or second group—to earn an A or a B, to my way of thinking.

I scored a big fat paniagua D. Oh, I kept up for a while, but when the race got serious, I got dusted and finished in the middle of the pack, the fourth group, fifteen minutes back. Meanwhile, Marty stayed with the first group most of the day, and finished in the second group—right in the mix. After the race, I felt a new level of frustration as I watched the white bags get handed out. Now I could measure the injustice. Marty used to be a few groups behind me; now he was a few groups ahead. I could count the number of seconds those white bags contained. I could see the gap between who I was and who I could be. Who I was supposed to be.

This was bullshit.

This was not fair.

In that moment, the future became clear. Unless

something changed, I was done. I was going to have to find a different career. I began to get more stressed and angry. Not at Marty—after all, he was only doing what a lot of others were doing. He'd been given the opportunity, and he'd taken it. No, I felt angry at myself, at the world. I was being cheated.

A few days later, I heard a soft knock on my door. Pedro walked in and sat down on the bed; we were knee to knee. His eyes were sympathetic.

"I know how hard you work, Tyler. Your levels are low, but you push yourself to keep up."

I acted tough, but he could tell how much I appreciated hearing that. He leaned in close.

"You are an amazing rider, Tyler. You can push yourself to the limit, even when you are completely empty; very few people can do this. Most riders, they would abandon. But you keep going."

I nodded. I could feel where he was going, and my heart started beating faster.

"I think you perhaps have a chance to make the Tour de France team. But you have to be healthier. You have to take care of your body. You must make yourself healthier."

The next day, I took my first EPO shot. It was so easy. Just a tiny amount, a clear liquid, a few drops, a pinprick on the arm. It was so easy, in fact, that I almost felt foolish—that was it? This was the thing I'd feared? Pedro gave me a few vials of EPO to take home along with some syringes. I wrapped it all up in foil and put it in the back of the fridge and, soon after, showed it to Haven. We talked about it for a few minutes.

"This is the exact same result as sleeping in an altitude

tent," I said. That wasn't completely true, of course, first because sleeping in a low-oxygen enclosure, or altitude tent (a legal method of boosting hematocrit) is a big hassle and gives you a headache, and also because it doesn't improve your blood values nearly as much. But the reasoning sounded good enough for both of us. We knew this was a gray area, but we also knew that the team doctor thought it was a good idea, for my health. We knew we were breaking the rules. But it felt more like we were being smart.

Besides Haven, I didn't talk about my decision with anyone. Not Scott, or Darren, or George, or Marty. They might've been like family, but telling them would've felt weird, like I was breaking a team rule. Now, I can see that the real reason I didn't want to tell was that I was ashamed. But back then, it felt like I was being savvy. I was becoming, in the word the Europeans liked to use, professional.*

---

* Hamilton's 1997 decision to start using EPO may have been based on an inaccurate assumption about his teammate, Marty Jemison.

"That spring, Tyler and I were in the same boat, hanging on by our fingernails," Jemison says. "I raced clean through the spring. Then in June, just before the Dauphiné, Pedro [Celaya] came to me and said if I was going to make the Tour team, I needed to be healthy. He taught me, he provided everything. So yeah, I did what the others did, starting in June and then in the Tour. But my Liège result was an honest result. I just had a good day."

Jemison, who won the U.S. national championship in 1999, rode just two Tours for Postal, a fact that might be attributed to the way the EPO era changed how teams assessed riders' potential. "I had a natural hematocrit of 48, so EPO didn't add that much horsepower to me," he says. "The longer I was [at Postal], the more I saw that I was no longer being groomed for the A team. Clearly, they were looking for riders who could deliver a whole new level of results." Jemison left the team after the 2000 season.

★ ★ ★

A lot of people wonder if taking EPO is risky to health. I'd like to reply to that concern with the following list:

Elbow
Shoulder
Collarbone (twice)
Back
Hip
Fingers (multiple)
Ribs
Wrist
Nose

Those are the bones I've broken during my racing career. This is not an unusual list in our profession. It's funny: in the States, everybody connects bike racing with health. But when you get to the top level, you see the truth: bike racing is not a healthy sport in any sense of the word. (As my former teammate Jonathan Vaughters likes to say, If you want to feel what it's like to be a bike racer, strip down to your underwear, drive your car 40 mph, and leap out the window into a pile of jagged metal.) So when it comes to the risks of EPO, they tend to feel pretty small.

What does being on EPO feel like? It feels great, mostly because it doesn't feel like anything at all. You're not wiped out. You feel healthy, normal, strong. You have more color in your cheeks; you're less grumpy, more fun to be around. These little clear drops work like radio signals—they instruct your bone marrow to create more red blood cells (RBCs), and soon millions more are filling up your veins, carrying oxygen to your muscles. Everything else about your body is the same, except now you have better fuel. You can go harder, longer. That holy place at the edge of your limits gets nudged out—and not just a little.

Riders talked of an EPO honeymoon, and in my experience it was true—as much a psychological phenomenon as anything else. The thrill comes from the way a few drops of EPO allow you to break through walls that used to stop you cold, and suddenly there's a feeling of new possibility. Fear melts. You wonder: How far could I go? How fast can I ride?

People think doping is for lazy people who want to avoid hard work. That might be true in some cases, but in mine, as with many riders I knew, it was precisely the opposite. EPO granted the ability to suffer more; to push yourself farther and harder than you'd ever imagined, in both training and racing. It rewarded precisely what I was good at: having a great work ethic, pushing myself to the limit and past it. I felt almost giddy: this was a new landscape. I began to see races differently. They weren't rolls of the genetic dice, or who happened to be on form that day. They didn't depend on who you were. They depended on *what you did*—how hard you worked, how attentive and professional you were in your preparation. Races were like tests, for which you could study. Instantly, my results began to improve; I went from getting C's and D's to getting A's and B's. As the summer began, I started figuring out the rules of the game:

1. Take red eggs for recovery once every week or two; make sure not to take them too close to races.
2 Get EPO at races, from the team doctors. You don't buy it; try to avoid keeping it in your house, except in special situations (like injury, or a long break between races). You inject it subcutaneously, into the fat layer beneath the skin. That helps it release more slowly, and provides a sustained effect.
4.Be quiet about it. There was no need to talk, because everybody already knew. It was part of being cool. Besides, if any laws were being broken, it was clear that the team was the one doing the breaking—they were the ones obtaining and distributing the EPO; my only job was to close my mouth, extend my arm, and be a good worker.

As the summer heated up, I started delivering real results, finishing in the top twenty, the top ten. I felt less tense, more relaxed. When other riders joked about their hematocrit numbers, I laughed along. I smiled knowingly when someone made a joke about EPO. I was the newest member of the white-bag club.

In June, we got the big news that Tour de France organizers had decided to invite Postal to the race. Then, a few weeks later, I got even bigger news when I was selected for the Tour team: I would be riding alongside Eki, George, Baffi, Robin, and the rest of the A team. I phoned my parents back in Marblehead and told them to fly over to watch part of the race. After all, this might never happen again. I was ecstatic—at least until the race began.

The 1997 Tour was crazily difficult. Normally, Tour stages are tough, but this year the organizers, perhaps reacting to the increased speed of the peloton, decided to make them *really* tough—one stage was 242 kilometers through the heart of the Pyrenees; seven continuous, camera-friendly hours of suffering. As a bonus, the weather was hellacious, featuring freezing rain, fog, and hurricane-strength winds. If the organizers were looking for a way to inspire EPO use, they succeeded. Postal went through a lot of white bags, and I'm sure we weren't alone.

A lot of people wonder why doping seems more prevalent at the longer, three-week races like the Tour de France. The answer is simple: the longer the race, the more doping helps—especially EPO. The rule of thumb: If you don't take any therapy in a three-week race, your hematocrit will drop about 2 points a week, or a total of about 6 points. It's called sports anemia. Every 1 percent drop in hematocrit creates a 1 percent drop in power— how much force you can put into the pedals. Therefore, if you ride a grand tour paniagua, without any source of red blood cells, your power will drop roughly 6 percent by the end of the third week. And in a sport where titles are often decided by power differentials of one-tenth of a percentage point, this qualifies as a deal breaker.

EPO or no EPO, the Tour's hardest day came on stage 14. On that day the French Festina team performed a circus strongman act the likes of which nobody had ever seen. At the foot of the 21.3-kilometer Col du Glandon, all nine Festina riders rode to the front, then went full bore, revving to unimaginable speed and carrying that speed over the climb of the Madeleine and into Courchevel. Later, we all realized what was happening: Festina was playing a new card. Something that went beyond EPO. Over the next day or so, the rumor circulated that Festina was using something called perfluorocarbons, synthetic blood that increases oxygen-carrying capacity, and for which there was no test. Using PFCs held huge, potentially life-threatening risks. The following year, a Swiss rider named Mauro Gianetti had ended up in intensive care; doctors suspected he'd used PFCs, though Gianetti denied it. But as Festina had shown, there were also rewards—which meant that these innovations, too powerful to stay secret for long, were quickly matched by other teams. "Arms race" is an accurate way to describe it, but it's important to realize that it was an arms race between teams, not individuals. Team doctors were trying to stay ahead of other team doctors; the riders' job was simply to be obedient.*

I rode the 1997 Tour, and survived. Riis was heavily

* Excessive displays like Festina's tended to occur whenever a new doping innovation appeared. They'd happened most notably in the spring of 1994 at the Flèche Wallonne race, when three Gewiss riders simply rode away from the rest of the field at an unthinkable speed. In the cycling world, this type of team domination had never happened before; it was the equivalent of an NFL team winning a playoff game 99–0. In addition, seven of the race's top eight finishers were all Italian, demonstrating that EPO innovation, like the Renaissance, began in Italy and traveled outward.

After the race, Gewiss team doctor Michele Ferrari was asked by a journalist if his riders used EPO. "I don't prescribe the stuff," he said. "But you can buy EPO in Switzerland without a prescription, and if a rider does, it doesn't scandalize me." When the journalist pointed out that numerous riders had died from using EPO, Ferrari said, "EPO is not dangerous; it's the abuse that is. It's also dangerous to drink ten liters of orange juice."

favored to win, but to the world's surprise, he was surpassed by a teammate, a wide-eyed, muscled twenty-three-year-old German named Jan Ullrich. Ullrich was a genuine phenomenon, with a fluid pedal stroke and incredible power for such a young rider. Watching him, I agreed with most observers: Ullrich was clearly Indurain's successor, the guy who was going to dominate the Tour for the next decade.

As for Postal, we did pretty well for a rookie team; our leader, Jean-Cyril Robin, finished 15th. I was 69th overall, the fourth Postie (Jemison was 96th, half an hour behind me; George was 104th). I wasn't the greatest rider in the world, but I was far from the worst. The new 50 percent hematocrit rule wasn't a big headache—in fact, I kind of liked it, since it seemed to reduce the frequency of strongman acts (there was still no test for EPO, remember). Thanks to the white bags and Pedro's spinner, it was easy to stay in the mid-forties. And if anybody on the team got too high, they could always lower their hematocrit by taking a speed bag—an IV bag of saline—or simply chugging a couple of liters of water and some salt tablets, a process we called "getting watered down."

In a Paris hotel after the Tour finished, I stood in front of a mirror and looked at my body. Slender arms. Legs with actual veins. Hollows in my cheeks I'd never seen before. A new hardness in my eyes. I went downstairs and met with the team and Thom Weisel and our sponsors. We raised champagne glasses and toasted the team's achievement. Weisel was pleased, but even then, with the bubbly in his hand, he was already talking about next year, when we'd *really* get it done.

By the spring of 1998 two of the Eurodogs had gone home, left the team. Scott had decided to go into the family business; Darren had decided to get a job in finance. George and I moved from the Dee-Luxe Apartment in the Sky to a modern three-bedroom apartment in the heart of Girona, near the Ramblas. We were sorry to see them go. They were good guys; we missed them. But we were also learning how our world worked. Some guys kept up; some didn't.*

* The commonsense question: If everybody was using EPO, then wasn't it just a level playing field? The answer, according to scientists, is no, because every drug affects different people differently. In the case of EPO, it is particularly illusory, due to the varying opportunities for improvement created by the UCI's 50 percent hematocrit limit.

For example: Hamilton's natural hematocrit is typically 42. Taking enough EPO to get to 50 means he could raise his hematocrit 8 points, an increase of 19 percent. In other words, Hamilton could add 19 percent more oxygen-carrying red blood cells—a huge increase in power—and still test under the hematocrit limit.

Now let's consider a different rider who has a natural hematocrit of 48. Under the 50-percent rule, that rider could only take enough EPO to add 2 points, or 4 percent more red blood cells—a power increase one-fourth of Hamilton's. That might be one of the reasons Hamilton's performance increased so rapidly when he started taking EPO.

Also, studies show that some people respond more to EPO than others; in addition, some people respond more than others to the increased training enabled by EPO. Then you have the fact that EPO shifts the performance limits from the body's central physiology (how much the heart pumps) to the peripheral physiology (how fast the enzymes in the muscles can absorb oxygen).

Bottom line: EPO and other drugs don't level the physiological playing field; they just shift it to new areas and distort it. As Dr. Michael Ashenden puts it, "The winner in a doped race is not the one who trained the hardest, but the one who trained the hardest and whose physiology responded best to the drugs."

Chapter 4

ROOMMATES

WHEN I HEARD LANCE was joining Postal for the 1998 season, I was excited and nervous. It made sense on paper—after all, we were the biggest American team, and Lance was the biggest American rider, or at least he had been before his illness. We'd all heard how he'd made it through the surgeries and the chemo, and over the last fourteen months, worked to get himself back into shape. We'd heard how he'd tried to get contracts from the big European teams; how Weisel had signed him for the relatively small amount of $200,000 plus bonuses. The question was, was Lance still Lance? Had cancer changed his abilities, his personality? We got the answer during the first day of training camp in California.

"Fuck you all!" Lance yelled as he took off, causing all of us to chase him. He was pretty strong, too—we had to work hard to bring him back.

"That all you fuckers got?" he asked when we caught him. "You pussies gonna let Cancer Boy kick your ass?"

I was relieved. I don't know what I was expecting—for Lance to show up whispering and bald, pushing a walker? He'd shed a few pounds—his arms no longer looked like a linebacker's—but otherwise he seemed utterly the same, with that same old aggression, that fists-up attitude.

When Lance enters a situation, he has a habit of shaking things up, raising the temperature of the room. I've come to believe that it's not something he can help: it's as though he's allergic to calm. It's almost like he's not comfortable unless there's a sense of discomfort, of intense and decisive action. He had a knack for seeking out weaknesses, for putting his finger on something that needs to be improved. He constantly judged everything: what kind of cereal we should have at the training table, where we should train, what kind of water bottle tops were best, which soigneur gave the best massage, where you could get the best bread, how to make espresso, what tech stock was going to take off—you name it, he knew it, and told you in no uncertain terms. Things he admired would earn an appreciative nod; things he didn't like would be dismissed with a puff of air through the lips: *phfffff* (a habit Lance seemed to have picked up from the Europeans). There were no gray areas; things were either amazing or awful. We used to joke that the one word guaranteed to piss Lance off was "maybe."

What Lance hated most of all, though, were choads. I'm not sure where the word came from—probably "chump" plus "toad"—but it meant what it sounded like. Choads were whiners, weaklings, guys who couldn't hack it or—worse—couldn't hack it and then complained. If you made a habit of being late or disorganized, you were a choad. If you weren't strong enough to ride in bad weather, or if you gave excuses for your performance, you were a choad. If you were a wheelsucker (someone who always rides in the slipstream of others), you were a choad. And once you were a choad, there was no going back.

Bobby Julich, for example. Bobby was a top American rider, one of Lance's old teammates on Motorola. I'm not sure why, but Lance never liked Bobby. Maybe it was because they'd competed against each other as juniors and remained rivals; maybe it was because Bobby could sometimes come across as Euro-sophisticated and intellectual (that kind of stuff never went over well with Lance), or because Bobby tended to hold forth about his latest injuries or his newest ideas about nutrition as if they were the most fascinating subjects in the world. Whenever Bobby's name came up, Lance would shake his head in that mix of disdain and disgust he used to signal the presence of a grade-A, certified choad. (To Bobby's credit, he didn't seem to care what Lance thought of him.)

Or Postal's director, Johnny Weltz. Johnny was a warm, friendly guy, but organization was definitely not his strong suit. Early in 1998 he screwed up a couple of times—I think it was arranging a hotel, or a race schedule, or equipment—and from then on, Lance was on the lookout for a new team director. That's a good measure of how much power Lance had at Postal: once he decided it, it was done. I'm not saying Lance was totally wrong— Johnny could be disorganized. But what was interesting, and sort of unimaginable to me, was the suddenness and completeness of Lance's decision, like some switch had been flipped. Just like that, Weltz was a choad, and was christened with a new name: Fucking Johnny Weltz. Whenever something went sideways, it was Fucking Johnny Weltz.

Fortunately for us, we also had two models for anti-choads: the tough Russian Viatcheslav Ekimov and our new teammate Frankie Andreu, one of Lance's Motorola teammates, who had signed with us. Lance didn't give his respect easily, but he respected Eki to the hilt—his work ethic, his professionalism, his ability to take on any challenge without blinking. Eki used to keep track of exactly how many kilometers he rode each year; sometimes we'd ask him the number just to hear it. Usually it was around 40,000 kilometers, enough to circle the earth.

Frankie was sort of our American Eki, and the closest thing Lance had to a big brother. No-Frills Frankie, you could call him: a big, strong, plainspoken Michigan guy, salt of the earth, who had everybody's respect. Frankie and Lance went way back; they'd ridden together on Motorola. On the bike, Frankie was a horse—he'd finished fourth in the 1996 Olympics, had a great nose for the attack. But it was off the bike that he had his real impact on the team, because he was one of the few who'd speak his mind, no matter what, especially to Lance. The soigneurs nicknamed Frankie "Ajax," after the blue scouring powder, because that was how it felt to talk with Frankie: you got scrubbed with the truth.*

---

* A year later, when Armstrong was late in paying the team the traditional bonuses after winning the 1999 Tour de France, Andreu went to Armstrong and reminded him to pay everyone their $25,000.

The truth wasn't pretty for Lance, at least at the beginning. He started out the 1998 season trying to ride as he had in the past—on training rides, he rode at the front of the group as much as he could, racing to stop signs, bombing down descents as if he were in a race. He pushed himself frantically, trying to show us and himself that he was back in shape. The problem was, he wasn't the same rider as before. His strength came and went unexpectedly. Some days he would be as strong as anyone. Other days it wasn't there; he'd disappear, pull off and go back to the hotel, become quiet and moody. You could tell the inconsistency was driving him crazy. He was fragile, viewing every day as a win or a loss, a triumph or a tragedy. There was no in-between.

The first race back in Europe was the Ruta del Sol in Spain, and Lance finished 15th. Afterward, the team congratulated him on the good finish, but Lance was having none of it. He wasn't sulking, exactly, but it was like he couldn't quite believe he hadn't won. He talks about how much he hates losing, but to me it's something deeper than hate. Losing short-circuits his brain: it's illogical; it's impossible. Like something in the universe is messed up, and it needs correcting. After that race, I think we all realized how big his ambition was, and how far he still had to go. I suppose I felt sorry for him.

That was the period when Lance and I started to spend more time together, both on and off the bike. I think Lance needed someone to talk to, to be with, and I was a good sounding board. Pretty soon we were riding next to each other on group rides, or grabbing a coffee. And not long after that, in the spring of 1998, we started rooming together at races. For me this was a huge honor, because I knew Lance had requested it.

I sometimes wonder why Lance picked me to room with, and I think it had something to do with the fact that I didn't kiss up to him as much as some guys did. You'd be surprised how much some people change their personalities around a guy like Lance—all of a sudden, people are talking louder, or showing off, or acting overly familiar with him. For example, I remember a lot of guys on the team called his wife, Kristin, by the nickname Lance used for her, "Kik," which made it sound like they were best buds—"I was hanging out with Lance and Kik yesterday," and the like. I never did that, because it felt too familiar. I always called Lance's wife Kristin, never Kik. You could call it politeness, or you could call it New England reserve; whatever it was, I got the sense that Lance appreciated it.

During the time we roomed together, Lance did almost all of the talking. He talked about each race at length, analyzing what went right and what went wrong. He nodded and *phffffff*-ed about the way the team was run, pointing out Johnny Weltz's lack of organization and applauding signs of progress. Most of all, Lance talked about other riders.

There's a type of conversation that happens (at least, used to happen in our era) between two teammates as they get to know each other. It's kind of strange: you both are doping, and you *know* you're both doping, but you never come out and say as much, at least at first. Instead, you talk about other people. You might say something like "That guy was flying." Or compare a rider to a motorcycle. Or say they were super-super-strong. The other racers know what you mean—they know you're talking about doping, and implying that the guy rode so fast because he was doped.

There was a phrase Lance used a lot during races: "Not normal." He'd say it whenever a rider was surprisingly strong. He said it in a loud, growling voice that was a bit jokey, but still meaningful. He said it loud, so everybody could hear. Sometimes he said it in French—*Pas normal*. For example:

A washed-up rider would make a solo breakaway, and win a big race—*not normal*.

A muscular sprinter would lead the pack up a long, steep climb—*not normal*.

A small, unknown team would suddenly have three finishers in the top ten—*not normal*.

After a while, I started saying it too. The words felt comforting, because they helped me ignore the fact that in our world, nothing was normal. Gradually Lance and I built some trust. We started to open up with each other a bit more, to talk shop. We talked about how much EPO we took at a time, how much of a boost we got (we were about the same). We talked about recovery products, our likes and dislikes. We talked about cortisone, which was used routinely in longer stage races to help combat fatigue and improve recovery (it was illegal, but if you had a therapeutic use exemption—basically a doctor's note— you could legally use it).

Lance told me how he sometimes felt blocked the day of a cortisone injection—meaning he couldn't really push himself as hard as he wanted—and how he preferred to take it the morning of an easier stage. He told me about bloatface, a reaction that happens when you take too much cortisone, and he reminded me of Ullrich in the final time trial of the '97 Tour—his face had been the size of a fucking pumpkin. Lance was an encyclopedia of information: he knew all the stories, even at races where he hadn't been. I had no idea how he stayed so connected, but man, he had sources. He constantly collected data on how other riders were training, what doctors they were working with, and what methods they favored, and he liked showing off his knowledge. I remember thinking that was strange—I only cared about my own program, not other people's.

"Fucking ONCE," Lance might say, referring to the Spanish team (pronounced UN-say) that finished first, second, and third at the Ruta del Sol. "First race of the year, and the whole team shows up fucking loaded to the gills. Fucking flying."

"Loaded to the gills" meant dope. We had a whole language: We called EPO "zumo," which is Spanish for "juice." We also called it "O.J.," "salsa," "vitamin E," "therapy," and "Edgar," which was short for Edgar Allan Poe. I can't remember who thought of that one, but we liked it: *Gonna speak with Edgar. Gonna visit Edgar. My old buddy Edgar.* If you overheard us talking you would have been excused for thinking that Edgar was a member of the team.

Lance would poke fun at the Spanish, but beneath was a thread of seriousness. He respected ONCE's team and their professionalism. They were a team that clearly had their program together. They had a fleet of experienced riders, good doctors, and a legendarily savvy director, Manolo Saiz. Lance wanted Postal to be more like ONCE.

But during the spring of 1998, it turned out, Lance had far bigger problems to deal with. At Paris–Nice, the season's first big race, Lance had a setback. It began with a disappointing prologue, and quickly multiplied when he ran into trouble in a freezing second stage. After spending a day chasing in the rain, Lance quit. He bailed. Did what we've all secretly wanted to do: he said screw it, pulled over to the side of the road, took off his race number, climbed into the team car, and flew home without telling anybody. Frankie saw it happen. He said he figured Lance was done with the sport.

I felt sad. I knew how much energy Lance had put into his comeback, how much he wanted it. I knew he'd be okay—there was no way Lance wasn't going to succeed at whatever he put his mind to. I could easily imagine him going to Wall Street, or running his own business, or going into broadcasting.

Then, after a few quiet weeks, we got the surprising news: it turned out Lance wasn't done. He was coming back across the Atlantic to give it one more try, at the Tour of Luxembourg in June. It wouldn't be an easy race. A boatload of top riders would be there: Erik Dekker, Stuart O'Grady, Erik Zabel, and Francesco Casagrande— guys gunning for the Tour de France. Nobody said it out loud, but the stakes were clear: this might be Lance's last shot. If he didn't do well in Luxembourg, his comeback might be over.

Lance and I roomed together in Luxembourg. We were in a cheap hotel, a cramped room with two twin beds. It was like we were two kids at sleep-away camp. Lance was on his bed, lying on his side, elbow crooked beneath his head. He started asking questions.

"So do you think I can beat Casagrande?" he asked.

—Sure.

"*Really?*" His voice went up.

—He can climb, but you'll kill him in the time trial.

"I'll kill him in the time trial," he repeated, as if memorizing the words. "I'll fucking kill him in the time trial."

—No doubt. Not even a contest.

A few seconds passed. Then Lance spoke again.

"So do you think I can beat Dekker?"

You can crush Dekker, I said, and I laughed to show how much I meant it. Then, just as with Casagrande, we went one by one through the reasons why he would absolutely crush Erik Dekker.

In this way, we went through most of the top contenders, until it seemed we'd completely switched roles: I was the old vet; he was the kid racer, fragile and unsure. Then there was one more question. Lance looked me in the eye—just like that first time we spoke. But this time, for once, he wasn't interested in delivering a message. He was genuinely curious.

"Do you think I can win the Tour someday?"

I hesitated, because in truth, I didn't see that happening. Lance was good, but we both knew the Tour was another level entirely. I remembered how Indurain had crushed him in 1994, how he'd never contended for the overall in a three-week race, how he'd finished only one of the four Tours he'd attempted thus far.

—Sure. You're strong already. Wait until you get stronger.

"Really?"

He was suspicious. He said what he often said: he was worried about his climbing.

—Look, you can climb with all those guys. Maybe not attack, but you can hang. You can time-trial with them. If you can hang on the climbs and time-trial, you can win. So I say, Yeah, you can win the Tour.

"You're not fucking with me. You think I can win the Tour."

—Definitely.

The interesting part was, I think Lance knew I was lying. His BS detector is top-notch. But in this case, he needed me to lie.

Seeing him like that, I could feel what he was up against. He had to win the physical battle—he had to get in race shape again. Then the strategic battle—he had to get a good team, one that would support him. Then, even if he did all that, he still had those strongmen like Riis and Casagrande out there, doing God knows what to beat him. I could see why he focused on the Tour. It was the biggest race in the world by far, the one goal that would be worth this immense effort.

The Tour of Luxembourg started well; Lance's form was coming around. Going into the last day he was tied for the lead. The weather was epically shitty, raining like hell and blowing sideways. Lance was stoked; he always preferred bad weather—not because he loved it, but because he knew it demoralized others.

I sometimes forget how much fun Lance was to race

with. He didn't go in with vague ideas, just hoping to do well. He was switched on, lit up from the inside; every move was life or death. When it didn't work, it was disaster—nothing could be worse. But when it worked, it was magic.

On the bus before the stage, Lance outlined the plan: we'd cover every single break, then attack on the steepest climb. It worked. Early in the stage, Lance, Marty Jemison, Frankie Andreu, and I made it into a small break-away, and we started gaining time on the field. Lance was screaming and yelling, going crazy. We'd left his competitors behind, but he still wanted more.

"Go go go go, fucking go! You guys are gonna earn some money today. You are gonna motherfucking get paid if we win this race."

Frankie, clever as always, made a late solo break and won the stage; we crossed the line a minute later, and Lance took the overall victory. As we crossed the finish line the loudspeakers were cranking Springsteen's "Born in the USA." Lance was lit up like a Christmas tree. He yelled, he whooped, he whacked us on the back. He phoned his agent, Bill Stapleton. He phoned Weisel. He phoned a *VeloNews* writer. He phoned his mom.

We won the race, we won the race, we won the race!

I liked the sound of that.

We.

To Lance's everlasting good fortune, he decided he wasn't ready to race the 1998 Tour de France and targeted the three-week Tour of Spain instead. He thus avoided having his comeback associated with the royal shitshow known as the Festina Affair. While he might have missed it, I didn't. I was riding my second Tour de France; it turned out to be one of the most memorable, and not in a good way.

It began when a Festina team car, driven by a Belgian soigneur named Willy Voet, got stopped and searched by French police at a border crossing. In the trunk was a stash of performance-enhancing drugs large enough to supply several pharmacies. Customs officers found 234 doses of EPO, 82 vials of human growth hormone, 160 capsules of testosterone, etc. (probably not a whole lot different from what Postal or many of the other teams were taking to the race). I remember being impressed that they were carrying hepatitis vaccine—pretty thoughtful, given how many shots those riders were getting.

The result: instant chaos. Gendarmes swarmed the Tour, searching team cars and buses. Festina team officials denied everything for a few days, then were kicked out of the race when the evidence became too great. Police raided Festina's offices and found a similar trove, including PFCs; it turned out the team maintained a slush fund for their dope to which riders were required to contribute the equivalent of a few thousand dollars each. The biggest surprise for me was when French riders got perp-walked—unlike in the U.S., doping is a crime in France. Riders staged dramatic but ultimately pointless protests, refusing to ride unless they were treated with respect. Meanwhile, teams were frantically flushing thousands of dollars' worth of pharmaceuticals down the toilets of buses, RVs, and hotels. I remember Ekimov joking that he was thinking about diving into the Postal team RV's toilet and pulling it out.*

The police didn't mess around. Alex Zülle, a Swiss contender who rode for Festina, was strip-searched, held in a cell for twenty-four hours, given nothing but one glass of water. He confessed: "Everybody knew that the whole peloton was taking drugs and I had a choice. Either I buckle and go with the trend or I pack it in and go back to my old job as a painter. I regret lying but I couldn't do otherwise."

I remember it was the one and only time I ever saw Pedro nervous. People were going to jail; in fact, Pedro's replacement at ONCE, a doctor named Terrados, was detained by the cops. I remember feeling strangely relieved at the whole thing. I knew I didn't have any EPO on me (well, in my veins perhaps, but there was no test yet). It felt weirdly good knowing that it'd be a level playing field, that we'd all be riding the rest of the Tour paniagua. I remember Frankie applying a little Ajax-style truth, saying that all this police craziness might be a good thing, that the sport was getting out of hand. We were only the foot soldiers in this messed-up arms race.

And beneath all the chaos, we heard rumors that a few riders did something that was either very brave or very stupid: they went to Plan B. They carried their own Edgar. They got it from other sources: quick dropoffs in hotel parking lots from girlfriends, mechanics, cousins, a

* In *From Lance to Landis*, by David Walsh (New York: Ballantine Books, 2007), Postal soigneur Emma O'Reilly says that she heard Postal staffers estimate that $25,000 in medical products was flushed down the toilet of the RV.

bartender friend of the coach. That's how it works. The authorities shut one door, riders open two windows.

In the wake of the busts, then, the 1998 Tour became a different sort of contest, less about who was the strongest, and more about who was the ballsiest, who had the best Plan B. And it turned out there were some good ones. The Polti team later confessed to keeping a thermos of EPO hidden inside a vacuum cleaner. The GAN team joked about stashing it by the side of the road. The race was won by Marco Pantani, the Italian climber, and dominated by the French team Cofidis, whose riders took three of the top seven spots, with none other than Bobby Julich finishing third. Cofidis's performance sparked rumors that the team had kept using EPO after the rest of the peloton had stopped; nothing was ever proven. The rest of us rode paniagua, dragged ass, survived.*

Amid all the controversy, I did manage to have a big moment, one that, when I look back, changed me. On July 18, the day after Festina was expelled, we rode the first true test of the Tour: a 58-kilometer individual time trial in Corrèze, a grueling course with a profile like shark's teeth. It was the kind of course built to favor big strong riders, not smallish guys like me. My team thought

---

* Cofidis's 1998 performance was statistically unusual. Over the rest of their careers, the top four Cofidis finishers (Julich, Christophe Rinero, Roland Meier, and Kevin Livingston) rode the Tour a collective fifteen times, averaging 45th place.

"It drove Lance crazy that Bobby [Julich] got third in the [1998] Tour," recalled Betsy Andreu, Frankie's wife. "Lance never considered Bobby to be that great of a rider, and so we used to tease Lance about it. Looking back, I think it motivated Lance a lot—if Bobby could get third, Lance probably figured he could win."

so little of my chances that they did not even send a team car to follow me in case I had a mechanical problem. This royally pissed me off, but I didn't say anything; I figured I'd let my legs do the talking.

And my legs didn't just talk—they sang. I pushed past my normal limits, felt myself pressing against that old wall, and—all of a sudden, I found another gear. I passed rider after rider; moving past them at speed. I pushed for the line, seeing stars from oxygen deprivation. When the stars cleared, I had beaten every single Tour de France rider except for one, the German wunderkind, Jan Ullrich. Observers were shocked. I was nearly as surprised as they were. Second place on the Tour's toughest day. Me.

That night, Pedro came to see me. He was twinkling; his eyes were shining with delight. More than anyone, he understood the deeper meaning of my result. There's a term they use in the sport, "revelation"—the ride where someone shows they have a champion's capacity. And Pedro informed me that I had just performed my revelation, and, more impressive, I'd done it with a hematocrit of only 44.

Forty-four! He said it several times. That number moved him, because in it he could see how fast I might have gone, might yet go if I became more professional. Then he put a fatherly hand on my shoulder, and he told me something that changed my life.

You can win the Tour de France someday.

I laughed out loud, told him to be quiet. But Pedro insisted. I could win the Tour. Not this year, not next year. But some year. He made the case with doctorly assurance.

*You can time-trial, you can climb, and you can push yourself
where no one else can. Listen and remember, Tyler. I know. I
have seen many, many riders, and you have something special,
Tyler. You are a special rider.*

I returned to the States when the season ended that fall. A
few months later, Haven and I got married. Occasionally,
over that off-season, the topic of doping would come up.
People had heard of the Festina Affair, and they wanted to
know what really happened. I usually responded by saying it was overblown, that there were a few bad apples
and now they'd been found out. I told people I was grateful for the scandal, because it helped the rest of us who
wanted to compete cleanly.

One afternoon, my father came to me with that
question. He sat me down; he brought up Festina. My
dad's a smart guy; he knew that Festina wasn't something
that could be brushed away. He was clear: he didn't want
me getting mixed up in a bad scene, in something I might
regret later.

I didn't hesitate.

"Dad, if I ever have to take that stuff to compete, I'll
retire."

I'd thought it would be hard to lie to my dad; it
turned out it was easy. I looked him right in the eye; the
words popped out so effortlessly that I'm ashamed to
think of it now. The truth was far too complicated to tell.
That fall, when other friends asked about Festina, I said
the same thing with even more conviction—*If I ever
have to take that stuff to compete, I'll retire.* Each time, the
words felt good to say. Each time, lying got easier.

They wanted to believe I was clean, and in a way, so did I.

When I spoke those words to my father, it sealed my life in bike racing behind a steel door. That was the moment I started learning what we all had to learn: how to live on two planets at once. Only Haven and I would know the real truth. And I knew, even as I assured my father everything was fine, that I was about to go in a lot deeper.

At the Postal banquet in Paris after the Tour, word had begun to go around the team. Given all the shit with Festina, teams weren't going to be able to keep supplying EPO and other products. Postal would pay for the legal recovery stuff, but beyond that, we were on our own. I understood the message loud and clear. A new era was about to begin.

Chapter 5

BAD NEWS BEARS

IT MAY NOT LOOK like it, but bike racing is the quint-essential team sport. The leader stands on the shoulders of his teammates—called domestiques, servants—who use their strength to shelter him from the headwind, set the pace, chase down attacks, and deliver water and food. Then, just out of sight, there's a second level of domestiques: the team director, the soigneurs, the mechanics, the drivers, the interconnected grid of people who are essentially doing the same thing. Every race is an exercise in cooper-ation—which means that when it goes well, it creates a kind of high like I've never felt anywhere else; a feeling of connectedness and brotherhood. All for one, one for all.

The 1999 Postal team was one of my favorite teams of all the ones I've ever been on. Not because of the remark-able things we accomplished together, but because of the extreme amount of fun we had while we were doing it. Now, looking back, I have mixed feelings about the methods we used to win the Tour. But I can't pretend that being on this particular team was anything but a complete blast because (1) Postal didn't do anything that other smart teams couldn't have done, and (2) we had absolutely nothing to lose.

We had Frankie Andreu. The field general, the road captain, with his gravelly Ajax voice you could hear from a hundred yards away. We had my Girona roommate, George Hincapie, the Quiet Man, who was maturing into one of the strongest riders in the world.

We had Kevin Livingston, newly signed from Cofidis, who was the engine, both socially and on the bike. Kevin was a brilliant climber, and an equally brilliant comedian. I've seldom laughed harder than when Kevin and I went out for beers—he could do dead-on impressions of everyone on the team (including Lance, though he wisely kept that one under wraps). During races, though, Kevin had a serious ability to "bury himself," that is, to push himself to his breaking point and past it, in the service of a teammate, especially when that teammate was Lance. Kevin's relationship with Lance went way back: when Lance was recovering from chemo treatments, Kevin had been the one to take him for his first rides.

We had Jonathan Vaughters, the Nerd. If Bill Gates had decided to become a cyclist, he might've been like Jonathan. Genius-level smart and naturally talented, Jonathan was known on the team for four things: (1) his ability to climb; (2) his incredibly messy hotel rooms, which looked like a laundromat had exploded in them; (3) his even-more-incredible gas, caused by the protein shakes he was constantly drinking; and (4) his tendency to ask uncomfortable questions, especially when it came to doping. While the rest of us simply did what the team doctors told us to do, Jonathan read books on sports science and designed his own training programs. He was always probing: Where did this stuff come from? What does it do? He was visibly more nervous about doping than the rest of us, but he was certainly no teetotaler: in fact, he set the record for climbing Mont Ventoux, one of the sport's toughest, most legendary peaks.

We had Christian Vande Velde, an easygoing, immensely talented Chicago kid whose claim to fame, besides being strong as hell, was that his father, John Vande Velde, played one of the evil Italian cyclists in the classic movie *Breaking Away* (some of the guys could recite the lines by heart). Christian was twenty-three, in his second year in Europe, and was taking everything in with wide-open eyes; he reminded me a little bit of me.

We had Peter Meinert Nielsen from Denmark and Frenchman Pascal Deramé, two big motors for the flats, and two good-natured guys. We had a crackerjack team of soigneurs, including Emma O'Reilly from Ireland and Freddy Viane from Belgium, who were whip-smart and funny to boot.

Then we had another type of teammate: the invisible kind. The person nobody talks about, but who is perhaps more important in the long run. That's where Motoman and Dr. Michele Ferrari come in. I met them around the same time, in the spring of 1999, during the run-up to the Tour.

I met Motoman at Lance and Kristin's villa in Nice, France, on May 15, just after I flew in from Boston. His first name was Philippe—I never learned his last name. He was trimming the rosebushes. I remember he wielded the garden shears carefully, as if he were performing some crucial task. Philippe was a slender, muscular guy with close-cropped brown hair, a broad forehead, and a gold earring. He had that French coolness that said, *Whatever you might say or do, I won't be surprised in the least.*

Lance gave me a quick rundown on Philippe's résumé: former amateur rider for a French team. Buddy of Sean Yates, a British rider and friend of Lance. Worked as a mechanic at a nearby bike shop. Philippe knew the local roads like the back of his hand; could show us all the best climbs. Lance had hired Philippe to take care of their place while they were gone, run errands, do odd jobs. Philippe was clearly proud of his status, but at the time it seemed Lance was the proud one, proud that he knew this cool French dude. Coolest of all, Philippe had a kick-ass motorcycle. I saw it when Philippe left: it was one of those crotch rockets, glossy and dangerous looking.

Kristin came outside and greeted us; she was four months pregnant. They'd recently purchased the villa, which looked like it had cost a pretty penny. It wasn't surprising to see Lance living large; he'd made big money before his cancer, and he knew how to spend it. Around us, workmen were finishing up the renovation, missing deadline after deadline in the traditional style.

Fuckin' French, Lance said.

To my eye, though, the place looked like something out of a movie. Rose garden, swimming pool, marble balconies from which you could look out on the red-tiled roofs of Nice and beyond to the blue Mediterranean.

Seeing them, I felt a twinge of wistfulness; Lance and Kristin were building a life, like the one Haven and I sometimes dreamed about. We had agreed that we didn't want to have kids, not yet, until things were more settled, and our tastes ran closer to cottages than villas. But some-day, definitely.

Right now, though, my concern was the immediate future. I'd been in Boston the previous two weeks, with zero access to our friend Edgar (at this point in my career, I wasn't about to risk taking it through customs, and had no sources of stateside EPO). As a result, my hematocrit was down, and I needed a boost, especially if we were about to train hard. When Kristin walked off, I turned to Lance.

—Hey dude, you got any Poe I can borrow?

Lance pointed casually to the fridge. I opened it and there, on the door, next to a carton of milk, was a carton of EPO, each stoppered vial standing upright, little soldiers in their cardboard cells. I was surprised that Lance would be so cavalier. On the occasions I had kept EPO in my Girona fridge, I had taken it out of its cardboard packaging, wrapped it in foil, and put it in the back, out of sight. But Lance seemed relaxed about it. I figured he knew what he was doing. I took a vial, and thanked him.

I needed to be on top of my game, because the next few weeks looked busy. Postal had undergone a Lance-driven makeover, adopting a Tour-first mentality. Team direc-tor Johnny Weltz had been replaced by Lance's handpicked choice: a sharp-eyed, just-retired Belgian rider named Johan Bruyneel. Johan had an ideal pedigree:

he'd ridden for the Spanish geniuses at ONCE and knew their system. Johan had the same savvy, information-driven mind as Lance did; from the start, the two were finishing each other's sentences. The overhaul meant new staff; Pedro's replacement was ONCE's former doctor, a humorless, overcaffeinated man from Valencia named Luis Garcia del Moral, whom the riders quickly nicknamed the Little Devil, or El Gato Negro (the black cat). Del Moral's harshness was balanced a little by the friendly, easygoing personality of his assistant, Pepe Martí.

There were other changes, too. Under the new, post-Festina system, we no longer got EPO from team staffers at races; instead we had to pick it up ourselves. I got it at del Moral's clinic in Valencia; some of my teammates drove to pharmacies in Switzerland, where it was sold over the counter. In theory, the new system was "for safety"—to avoid a repeat of the Festina Affair. But to me it was the opposite, because now the risk of transport and border crossing was ours, to say nothing of the expense. I didn't like it, because it was yet another thing to deal with, another chore. But I did it. On May 25, I drove to Valencia and picked up 20,000 units—a couple months' worth—for around $2,000.

More urgently, we had six weeks left before the start of the Tour de France, and we were facing a bunch of questions, the biggest of which was whether Lance would be strong enough to contend. Would the team be strong enough to support him? And, in the back of our minds, one more question: Would we risk bringing Edgar along during the race? Carrying EPO in the team vehicles was out of the question. Yet, as we knew from the previous year, any rider or team who had access to EPO during the race would have a tremendous advantage.

That's where Philippe came in.

We were standing in Lance's kitchen when he lined out the plan: he would pay Philippe to follow the Tour on his motorcycle, carrying a thermos full of EPO and a prepaid cell phone. When we needed Edgar, Philippe would zip through the Tour's traffic and make a dropoff. Simple. Quick—in and out. No risk. To be discreet, Philippe wouldn't be supplying all nine of us; it would just be the climbers, the ones who needed it most and would provide the biggest bang for the buck: Lance, Kevin Livingston, and me.* Los Amigos del Edgar. From that moment on, Philippe wasn't Philippe the handyman anymore. Lance, Kevin, and I called him Motoman.

Lance practically glowed when he told me about the plan—he loved this kind of MacGyver secret-agent stuff. Aside from Johan Bruyneel, we three would be the only ones who knew. The French could search us all day long and they'd find zero. And besides, we felt sure that most of the other teams would be doing their own version of Motoman. Why wouldn't they? Lance had come back from cancer; he wasn't about to sit back and hope things worked out; he was going to make it happen. He was incapable of being passive, because he was haunted by what others might be doing. This was the same force that drove him to test equipment in the wind tunnel, to be

* Livingston has never commented publicly on doping matters. He did not respond to interview requests.

finicky about diet, to be ruthless about training. It's funny; the world always saw it as a drive that came from within Lance, but from my point of view, it came from the outside, his fear that someone else was going to out-think and outwork and outstrategize him. I came to think of it as Lance's Golden Rule: *Whatever you do, those other fuckers are doing more.*

That rule was why Lance worked with the other in-visible Postal teammate, Dr. Michele Ferrari. Ferrari was a forty-five-year-old Italian doctor with a reputation for being so brilliant, so innovative, that he'd single-handedly reshaped the sport. He'd worked for the biggest riders and teams, he charged the biggest fees, and he was so mysterious that in the peloton he was known as "the Myth."

I met Ferrari for the first time in April 1999, at a rest stop by the side of the highway that runs between Monaco and Genoa, Italy. Ferrari showed up, a skinny, bespectacled, birdy-looking guy, driving a humble camper. At first it seemed kind of a letdown. Given Ferrari's reputation (not to mention his name), I'd expected to see him arrive in a sleek Italian sports car. Only with time did I realize how brilliant this was; the perfect camouflage.

Ferrari was unlike any other doctor I'd ever met, before or since. While Pedro was all about the human connection, Ferrari approached you like you were an algebra problem that needed solving. He traveled with his own scale and skin-fold calipers for measuring body fat. He had a hematocrit spinner, syringes, and a calculator. He looked at me with those dark eyes through oversize 1980s glasses, and I could almost hear the numbers whirring in his head. Unlike Pedro, Ferrari couldn't have cared less about how you were feeling, or what was happening in your life. He was interested only in body weight, fat percentage, wattage (the measure for power—basically how much force you put into the pedals), hematocrit. I was hoping to impress him with my fitness; after all, in six days we'd be racing 257-kilometer Liège–Bastogne–Liège, one of the spring's toughest tests. But when Ferrari analyzed me, he shook his head in disappointment.

Ahhh, Tyler, you are too fat.

Ahhh, Tyler, your hematocrit is only 40.

Ahhh, Tyler, you don't have enough power.

Whatever, I thought. Then he said something else.

Tyler, you will not finish Liège.

The hell I won't, I thought. Ferrari's certainty angered me. I wasn't just some equation. How could he know what I was capable of? As it turned out, Ferrari was wrong. I did finish Liège—in fact, I finished 23rd, my best finish to date, and I thought about Ferrari the entire race.

But Lance loved Ferrari. Ferrari appealed to his love of precision and numbers and certainty. I got the feeling that Lance's relationship with Ferrari was like mine with Pedro: complete trust. It was clear that Ferrari had told Lance if he hit certain numbers, he had a chance to win the Tour de France. This idea ignited Lance. It gave him the kind of specific target he thrived on. In the months before the Tour, we trained harder than I'd ever trained. Lance focused on Ferrari's promise: hit the numbers and good things will happen.*

Ferrari's importance in Lance's life was pretty obvious, mostly because Lance talked about him all the time, especially while we trained. Ten people could give him the exact same piece of advice, but if it came from Michele, it was gospel. My understanding was that Lance valued Ferrari so much that he had worked out an exclusive agreement that Ferrari would not train any other Tour contenders. Kevin and I used to say that Lance said the word "Michele" more often than he said the word "Kik."

Even so, Lance tried to keep his relationship with Ferrari quiet from the rest of the team—not always with success.

JONATHAN VAUGHTERS: I remember one time during [the Spanish race] Setmana Catalana in March 1999. Marco Pantani totally dominated the first climbing stage; he was flying, looking really good, and Lance was in the middle of the pack. At the finish, we get into the team car and right away Lance is on his cell phone having this really intense

---

* The reverse was also apparently true: if his numbers were off, Armstrong got nervous—a point that was underlined in January of 1999 at Postal team training camp in Solvang, California. The whole team rode a 10-kilometer time trial, and then had their blood tested afterward; the blood values and the time were combined into an overall fitness score. When the scoring was done, Lance was second—Christian Vande Velde was first. But rather than tell Lance, Bruyneel tweaked the result slightly so that Lance finished first. As George Hincapie told *New York Times* reporter Juliet Macur: "We didn't want to tell Lance because it would have upset him, but no one ever told Christian, either. We kind of didn't want to upset the hierarchy."

conversation with someone about what he needs to do to go faster than Pantani three months from now at the Tour. But it's not a normal conversation, because Lance is talking in code. I don't remember the precise wording, but it was something like "Should I take one apple this week or two apples next week?" Then Lance hangs up the phone and I ask, "Who was that?" And Lance says, "None of your business." Later, I put two and two together; it had to be Ferrari.

Looking back now, it's kind of amazing to realize how many different random factors lined up in our favor in the 1999 Tour de France. It's even more amazing when you think about how important the 1999 Tour turned out to be in the whole scheme of things; how it got the wheels turning for the whole crazy ride that came afterward. What's still more amazing—what I still sometimes lie in bed thinking about, almost fifteen years later—is how close it all came to not happening at all.

On July 3, we headed to the Tour de France prologue, and it wasn't hard to tell which team was the underdog. Around us, teams like ONCE, Banesto, and Telekom had rock-star buses with couches, halogen lighting, stereo systems, TVs, showers, and espresso machines.

We, on the other hand, were the Bad News Bears. We had two of the crummiest family campers on the Continent. One was rented; the other belonged to Julien DeVriese, Postal's crotchety Belgian head mechanic. We called it Chitty Chitty Bang Bang, because everything shook when you drove: the cabinet doors tended to fly open on the gentlest curve; every hinge squeaked frantically; it was so loud that, when under way, you could barely talk over the din. Julien had one rule: *No shitting in the camper*. He was very clear on this rule. We could tell because every time we saw him, he would point his big finger at us and say, "No shitting in the campa!" in a husky voice. We informed Julien that shitting in the camper was likely to improve it.

I couldn't complain, though, because I was lucky enough to be assigned to the better camper. It was better because we had only three riders in ours—Lance, Kevin, and myself, plus a driver. The worse camper held the other six Postal team members, who were crammed in like college kids in a phone booth. The logic behind our seating chart was Motoman: Lance, Kevin, and I would be the only team members to get EPO during the race, so it made sense that the Amigos del Edgar should have our own space. Cleaner that way, as Lance put it. We kept it secret, but the other guys knew something was up.

Despite the campers, we had a growing good feeling about the race. During the run-up to the Tour, it seemed every week brought another piece of news about Tour de France contenders.

- Back in January, the French cycling federation had started testing the blood profiles of their riders; it was called longitudinal testing, and it basically meant that it would be harder for the French to take EPO and get away with it.
- In May, Belgian star Frank Vandenbroucke was suspended for buying drugs.

- In June, on the brink of winning his second Tour of Italy, 1998 Tour de France winner Marco Pantani, the best climber in the world and one of the guys Lance feared most, was suspended for exceeding the 50 percent hematocrit rule.

- In mid-June, the German magazine *Der Spiegel* published an investigative report detailing organized doping on Telekom, the largest German team, home to both Bjarne Riis and Jan Ullrich. The article was filled with details, including training plans (they called EPO "Vitamin E," and paid a lot less than we did—about $50 for 1,000 units, while we paid closer to $100). The article spoke of Telekom's use of a private clinic; it quoted team trainers who vouched that Riis had raced the 1995 Tour—one he *didn't* win—with a hematocrit of 56.3. We read about the report and the ensuing controversy, and felt a mix of emotions: on one hand, fear that such details could emerge; on the other, relief that we didn't have the pressure and attention of being a big European team.

- In late June, both Riis and Ullrich suffered injuries at the Tour of Switzerland—a broken elbow for Riis, and a knee injury for Ullrich—that would keep them out of the Tour.

All that added up to make the 1999 Tour one of the most wide-open fields in modern history, the first in fifty years without a former winner in the lineup. Lance was on a long list of hopefuls behind Alex Zülle (the now-former Festina rider who was allowed to return after a brief ban and fine), French favorite Richard Virenque (ditto), Spanish climber Fernando Escartín, Italians Ivan Gotti and Wladimir Belli, and Bobby Julich. Tour organizers did their best to dress up the situation, calling the 1999 race the "Tour of Renewal."

Like most people, I figured Lance's chance of winning was small, mostly because he had yet to prove that he could climb with the best. Also, I worried about the Motoman plan. Every time I saw a gendarme, I thought of Philippe, somewhere out there with the EPO and the phone. What if he got stopped? What if he decided to sell us out, to talk to police, the press? The Motoman plan suddenly felt like a huge, crazy gamble. But if Lance was worried, he didn't show it. He's never happier than when he's making a bet, moving one step ahead, playing chess. When I seemed worried, he would reassure me. *This is all going to work. It's foolproof. We're going to fucking throttle everybody.* Apparently Johan Bruyneel was confident as well.

JONATHAN VAUGHTERS: A few days before the Tour, I went up to Johan and asked him if the team was going to be carrying anything illegal into France. I'd seen what happened with Festina, and frankly I was scared shitless about getting arrested. So I ask Johan, "Our team isn't going to be bringing anything into France, right?" Johan smiles at me, this big knowing smile. He says, "You don't need to worry about anything."

The funny thing was, the Tour nearly ended before it began. A day or so before the race Johan informed us that, according to the Tour's medical tests, several of our hematocrits were dangerously close to surpassing the 50 percent limit: I don't remember all the exact numbers, but they were all in the high forties. George was 50.9 (back then you only got dinged if you went *past* 50; the threshold was later reduced to 50.0). None of us were over, but we were awfully close, and it didn't look good in the eyes of the UCI. I remember Jonathan Vaughters being particularly worried. We set about correcting the situation in the usual way: taking salt tablets and chugging as much water as we could hold. Jonathan said he peed every two hours that night.

Then, another near miss. The day of the prologue, we were previewing the 6.8-kilometer course for the final time. Lance was checking to see if he could climb the last hill in a big gear. He was on the flats going full blast, looking down at his chainring, when a Telekom team car pulled out right in front of him. Lance was on a path to smash directly into it at full speed. But George spotted the car and yelled, Lance looked up just in time to turn slightly. He got clipped by the mirror and knocked down, but was okay. I sometimes wonder what would've happened if George hadn't noticed, hadn't yelled.

Lance blazed the prologue, winning by seven seconds over Zülle. I think he was as shocked as the rest of the world was. He crossed the line, and didn't quite know what to do. The first person he hugged was the Little Devil, Dr. del Moral. In post-race interviews, Lance was charmingly stumbly and tongue-tied. He kept talking about how great this was for the team, for the staff, for everybody. It didn't feel real. It felt temporary—a fluke that would no doubt be corrected.

Two days later, the opposite happened. Stage 2 took us through Brittany and across the Passage du Gois, a narrow causeway that connects the island of Noirmoutier to the mainland, and which is only uncovered at low tide. Tour organizers love spectacular visuals, and so, about 80 kilometers into the ride, we found ourselves racing like hell across the causeway, which was wet and slick. Lance and George had smartly battled their way to the front; the rest of us fought to follow them in case of a crash. Sure enough, early in the crossing, someone in the middle of the pack wiped out; the ensuing demolition-derby pileup sent dozens of riders flying, blocked the road, and took Jonathan Vaughters out of the race. Most of the other contenders—including Zülle, Belli, and Gotti—were stuck behind the crash. They remounted in a panic and tried to catch up, but it was futile.

Just like that, Lance had a colossal six minutes on his main rivals. People spoke of it as luck, but that's not how we saw it within the race, and certainly not how Lance saw it. Everybody knew the causeway was going to be slick. Everybody knew that crashes were likely. Everybody had a chance to get to the front. It was the same with everything: the unfairness was part of what made the Tour fair, because everybody had to deal with it. You made it or you didn't. Period.

But the Tour was far from over. Everybody knew the key stages were 8 and 9: a 56-kilometer time trial in Metz, followed by a rest day, then the queen stage—a wicked triple-header of climbs of the Télégraphe, Galibier, and a mountaintop finish in the Italian ski village of Sestrière. As we rolled toward the showdown, the media used the week to whip up the plotlines, most of which revolved around a couple of questions: Was the peloton truly clean? Would Lance, who'd never been great on the long European climbs (his only Tour finish in four attempts was 36th), be able to climb with the rest of the contenders?

A couple days before, we got prepared. We used the secret phone to call Philippe, who zipped through the crowds and made his delivery. Since we wanted to keep the EPO out of our hotel, we usually did the shots in the camper. It worked like this: we'd finish a stage, and go straight into the camper for cleanup, get a drink, and change clothes. The syringes would be waiting for us, sometimes tucked inside our sneakers, in our race bags.

The sight of the syringe always made my heart jump. You'd want to inject it right away—get it in you and then get rid of the evidence. Sometimes del Moral would give the shot, sometimes we'd do it ourselves, whatever was fastest. And we were fast—it took thirty seconds at most. You didn't have to be precise: arm, belly, anywhere would do. We got into a habit of putting our used syringes in an empty Coke can. The syringes fit neatly through the opening—*plonk, plonk, plonk*—you could hear the needles rattle. And we treated that Coke can with respect. It was the Radioactive Coke Can, the one that could end our Tour, ruin the team and our careers, maybe land us in a French jail. Once the syringes were inside, we'd crush it, dent it, make it look like trash. Then del

Moral would tuck the Coke can at the bottom of his back-pack, put on aviator sunglasses, open that flimsy camper door, and walk into the crowds of fans, journalists, Tour officials, even police, who were packed around the bus. They were all watching for Lance. Nobody saw the anonymous guy with the backpack, who walked quietly through them, invisible.

In the stage 8 time trial Lance did well, winning over Zülle by nearly a minute (I didn't do too badly, finishing fifth). But it was stage 9 that everybody was waiting for—the climb to Sestrière. The first big climb of the Tour is a coming-out party, the moment the race really begins. Everybody's watching because this is when the Tour contenders finally show their cards.

The morning was cold and rainy. The early part of the race brought lots of attacks; everybody was trying to prove himself. Frankie did a magnificent job as road captain, watching the potential breakaways like a hawk, making sure we didn't let any contenders get away. We protected Lance as long as we could, then fell back, leaving him with an elite group of contenders. A few long-shot guys broke away; then Escartín and Gotti, who were thought of as the best climbers, took off after them. The script of the race looked clear: Lance had done well, but now it was time for the real climbers to take over. Escartín or Gotti would most likely win.

Then, with about eight kilometers left, something unexpected happened: Lance attacked, rode down Escartín and Gotti, and soloed away to take the stage win. I knew Lance was going well; I could hear the roar ahead of me on the road, and I could hear Johan and Thom

Weisel shouting jubilantly over the team radio. But it wasn't until that night, when I saw the highlights on television, that I realized how strong Lance had been.

"Armstrong has just ridden across like they were standing still!" commentator Paul Sherwen shouted. Lance's attack on Escartín and Gotti was even more impressive because of the way he did it—not standing, as most attackers do, but sitting down. His cadence barely changed. He just kept riding, churning that gear, and the other riders fell away. I knew how strong Lance was—we'd trained next to each other, day after day. But this got my attention, just like it got everyone else's. This was a new Lance, one I hadn't seen before. He was on a different level.

The doubters started in immediately. We later heard that some old hands in the press room had laughed out loud when Lance made his winning move—not in admiration, but because they thought his doping was so obvious. The stories the next day were filled with accounts of Lance the "extraterrestrial," which is the code they use to describe a doped rider. The French newspaper *L'Équipe* said Lance was "*sur une autre planète*"—on another planet.

Then it got worse. The French newspaper *Le Monde* uncovered the fact that Lance had tested positive for cortisone after the prologue, which caused a small but intense shitstorm. Not just for Postal, but for the entire Tour, which could not afford another doping scandal. They had the perfect comeback story in Lance, who embodied the Tour's triumphant return from the dark cloud of the Festina Affair. Now everything was suddenly at stake.

Postal and Lance handled it in a simple way. They produced a cover story: they said Lance had a saddle sore, and, according to reports, backdated a prescription for a cortisone-containing skin cream.* Though the doubters pointed out that Armstrong had failed to account for the prescription on his pre-Tour medical form, nobody aside from a few journalists seemed to care. The UCI didn't want to catch Lance; they accepted the prescription, and the Tour of Renewal rolled on.†

That was when the Tour became a different kind of sport; one that was all about controlling the story, which meant controlling the journalists. In 1999, as in every other year, most Tour de France journalists wanted to focus on the drama and romance of the race and avoid the doping issue if possible. But not all of them. A small group was focused on asking tough questions. Armstrong called this second group the trolls. The game was simple: the trolls tried to drag Lance down, and he tried to fight them off.

At first, Lance wasn't very good at this game. He was

---

* As Postal soigneur Emma O'Reilly recounted in *From Lance to Landis*: "At one stage, two of the team officials were in the room with Lance. They were all talking. 'What are we going to do, what are we going to do? Let's keep this quiet, let's stick together. Let's not panic. Let's all leave here with the same story.'" O'Reilly says that after the meeting Armstrong told her, "Now, Emma, you know enough to bring me down."

† As far as the UCI goes, this kind of cooperation wasn't new. In his 1999 book, *Massacre à la chaîne*, published in English as *Breaking the Chain* (London: Random House, 2002), Festina soigneur Willy Voet says the UCI similarly accepted a backdated therapeutic use exemption for lidocaine to help French cyclist Laurent Brochard avoid a positive test at the 1997 world championships.

defensive, off balance, touchy. "It's been a week, and nothing's been found," he said in one interview, his voice rising too much. "You're not gonna find anything. If it's *L'Équipe*, if it's channel 4, if it's a Spanish paper, Dutch paper, Belgian paper, there's nothing to find." Another time, he pointed out: "I've never tested positive. I've never been caught with anything."

Never been caught with anything?

But Lance caught on fast. I remember at a press conference one journalist pointed out that many people found his success to be nothing short of a miracle. Did he see it that way? Lance, who's not religious, thought about it for two seconds, then delivered a genius answer.

"It *is* a miracle," Lance said. "Because 15 or 20 years ago I wouldn't be alive, much less starting the Tour de France or leading the Tour de France. So yes, I think it's a miracle."

When the trolls kept harping on the cortisone story, Lance did what he did best: he decided to take them on directly. He started by calling *Le Monde* (a newspaper with a sterling reputation) "the gutter press," and "vulture journalism." He beefed up his denials; instead of focusing on himself, he focused on the motives and credibility of his attackers. At one point in a press conference, when a reporter kept digging, Lance said, "Mr. Le Monde, are you calling me a liar or a doper?"

I couldn't imagine saying something like that, or what I would've said if the reporter had replied, "Actually, I'm calling you both." But Lance showed me the raw power of the pure attack. He pulled it off because he believed— still believes—that what he did wasn't cheating, because in his mind all the other contenders in the race were on cortisone, had their own version of Motoman, and everybody was doing everything they could to win, and if they weren't, then they were choads and didn't deserve to win.

I've always said you could have hooked us up to the best lie detectors on the planet and asked us if we were cheating, and we'd have passed. Not because we were delusional—we knew we were breaking the rules—but because we didn't think of it as cheating. It felt fair to break the rules, because we knew others were too.

Are you calling me a liar or a doper?

I think that was the moment when Lance started winning. He showed them he wasn't like the rest, he wasn't going to duck or mumble some half-assed denial and wait for the trolls to drag him down. And it worked. The stories in the next day's media cycle didn't dwell on suspicions or positive tests; instead they told of Lance's fight against these charges, a fight that couldn't help but remind people of Lance's fight to come back after his illness. He took on the doubters, just like he took on cancer, and it worked.

The writers weren't the only people Lance had to deal with, of course. There was also French rider Christophe Bassons. Bassons was an interesting guy: a massive natural talent (his VO_2 max—maximum oxygen consumption, a measure of aerobic capacity—was 85, two points higher than Lance's score) who not only refused to take dope, but broke omertà by speaking out openly against it. His teammates called him Monsieur Propre—Mister Clean. The real problem, from Lance's point of view, was that Bassons wouldn't keep his mouth shut. As he rode the

1999 Tour, Bassons was also writing a column for *Le Parisien* in which he was telling the truth: that the Festina Affair had changed nothing.

Lance decided to fix things. The day after his win at Sestrière, he rode up to Bassons during the race and told him that his comments were hurting the sport; Bassons replied that he was telling the truth; Lance suggested that Bassons go fuck himself, and that he should get out of the sport.

At this point, riders could have rallied to Bassons' side; spoken out. But for whatever reason—perhaps fear, perhaps the strength of Lance's personality, perhaps force of habit—they didn't. During the stage and the following day, it became clear that Bassons was isolated. No one defended him. No one would talk to him, not even on his own team. Bassons understood, and dropped out the following day.

Throughout all this controversy, we were coming together as a team. With Lance in the yellow jersey, we had to use all our strength to control the race. It got tougher. We'd already lost Jonathan; then we lost Peter Meinert Nielsen to severe tendinitis in his knee. Each day was the same: Johan would begin by outlining some difficult plan, usually one that called for us to control most of the race. Then Lance would give us a pep talk, and our hearts would fill up with the importance of this moment, with the sheer unlikeliness of us, the Bad News Bears in a couple of shitty campers, winning the biggest race in the world. And it worked: each day we would go bury ourselves, and keep Lance safely in yellow.

As the Tour wore on, the riders who did not have

access to Edgar took the brunt of it. They were riding stone-cold paniagua, and they were doing one heck of a job, so we looked for ways to help out. One night during the second week we found that we had some extra Edgar—a couple thousand units, maybe. What to do? We didn't want to throw it away, and we didn't want to risk pushing our hematocrits too high. Lance was the one who made the suggestion: give it to Frankie. Someone was dispatched to his room; it turned out that Frankie was so exhausted that he was already asleep. Frankie nodded wearily and accepted the offer.

With each passing day, we drew closer to the Paris finish. We tried not to think about winning; we tried to focus on containing Zülle and the other contenders. But on July 21, when we rode into the Pyrenean city of Pau with Lance's lead intact and the final mountain stage behind us, the possibility became real. Unless something went drastically wrong—a crash, illness, or injury— Lance would win the Tour de France.

The only bad news was that we'd heard that one of our team was cracking: Philippe. Motoman was exhausted. I felt for him: following the Tour day after day, week after week, must've been brutal. Crowds are immense. Roads are closed. Hotels are completely booked. So Philippe camped, bivouacked, improvised shelters in road stops and parking lots. On one of his phone calls to Johan or Lance, Motoman confessed he was cracking. He couldn't do it anymore. Fortunately, by now the race was safely in hand. With a week left, Motoman was told he could head home to Nice.*

Near the Tour's finish, Lance suggested to Kevin and

me that it would be nice if we found a way to thank Philippe for his hard work. We knew that Lance was buying Rolexes for some of the soigneurs and coaching staff, so Kevin and I decided to do the same for Philippe. We chipped in cash, and Kevin's fiancée, Becky, picked up the watch in Nice and carried it with her to Paris.

The last week went like clockwork; so smooth that when we finally clinched it, we couldn't quite bring ourselves to believe it. After crossing the finish line, we made that traditional ride down the Champs-Élysées, saw the Arc de Triomphe surrounded by a massive crowd waving American and Texas flags, got off our bikes and wandered around the cobblestones in happy disbelief, hugging our wives, our families, each other. I remember champagne

---

* In 2005, as part of a retrospective study by the Châtenay-Malabry French national doping-detection lab to improve their methods, urine tests from the 1999 Tour de France were tested for EPO. Using the six-digit rider identification number, *L'Équipe* reporter Damien Ressiot established that fifteen samples belonged to Armstrong. Of the fifteen samples, six tested positive for EPO, including those taken after the prologue, and stages 1, 9, 10, 12, and 14; in addition several others showed the presence of artificial EPO in levels too low to trigger a positive test. All samples taken after stage 14 tested negative.

Armstrong argued that the samples may have been tampered with. But according to Dr. Michael Ashenden, one of the world's foremost doping experts, the odds of someone successfully tampering with the samples to achieve this precise spiking and tailing effect would be beyond astronomical; in fact, he's not aware of any lab equipment that is calibrated to such a degree. As Ashenden summed up, "There is no doubt in my mind that [Lance Armstrong] took EPO during the '99 Tour."

Perhaps more interestingly, it looks as though Armstrong was in the minority in 1999. Of the eighty-one urine samples taken during the 1999 Tour that were not Armstrong's, only seven tested positive for EPO, or 8.6 percent.

bottles popping, a million flashbulbs going off, a guy in the crowd playing a tuba. It felt like we were inside a Hollywood movie.

The victory party was equally fantastic. Thom Weisel rented the top floor of the Musée d'Orsay, a Beaux-Arts museum on the banks of the Seine; about two hundred sponsors, family, and friends attended. Weisel was in his glory, toasting everyone in sight and reminding us that we had just won the Tour de Fucking France. I remember seeing Lance's agent, Bill Stapleton, on the balcony, making calls, making plans—Letterman, Leno, Nike, the *Today* show, you name it—his phone was flashing like Times Square. At one point during the party, Lance's cell phone rang. He stood up, took the call, and came back a few minutes later.

"That was cool," he said. "That was President Clinton."

It was a time to thank the people who made it all possible. Lance went to the podium and said, "I wore the maillot jaune onto the Champs-Élysées today but my responsibility for that was equal to just about the zipper. The rest of the body, the sleeves, the collar were there because of my team, the support staff, and my family. And I mean that from the bottom of my heart."

Amid all the craziness, over in a quiet corner of the hall, we made time for a private ceremony. Kevin and I presented a tired, happy Motoman with his Rolex, his reward for helping to make the victory possible. We gave him a hug, and he tried it on. It fit perfectly.

Chapter 6

2000: BUILDING THE MACHINE

YOU AND HAVEN should move to Nice.

Lance said it lightly, but it felt big. In the fall of 1999 I was still based in Girona, but it was clear that the team's center of gravity had shifted to Nice, that beautiful city in the heart of the French Riviera. Lance and Kristin lived there; so did Kevin Livingston and his now-wife, Becky, as well as Frankie Andreu and his wife, Betsy; Michele Ferrari was a half day's drive away. Haven had recently left her job at Hill Holliday so we could live together full-time in Europe. Living in Nice sounded better than perfect: all of us together, training, working, living, preparing for the next Tour. So, in March 2000, Haven and I moved into a small yellow house at the end of a rose-covered lane in Villefranche, about a mile from Lance and Kristin. We also, for the first time, had money: a new $450,000 contract (a healthy $300,000 increase from the previous year) plus a $100,000 bonus if I helped Lance win the Tour again.

It felt like moving to another planet: the billionaires' yachts bobbing in the harbor and the older French couples with enormous sunglasses and tiny dogs. From our new place we could see Nellcôte, the mansion where the Stones recorded *Exile on Main Street*; Monaco was just around the corner. It was the kind of place where you walked past a glamorous woman on the street, and one second later realized, *Whoa, that was Tina Turner*.

Kevin, Lance, and I. We rode together most days, with Frankie joining up some of the time. We'd usually meet on the road by the sea, then head up and out into the mountainous country north of Nice. Training like that is sort of like sitting with your friends and watching a movie—in this case, the movie was the countryside of France, scrolling past us. As with movies, you spend most of your time talking nonsense, making observations, trying to crack each other up.

We all had our roles. Frankie was the anchor: clear-eyed, unflappable. Kevin was the fizz; he was always bubbling with good humor, stupid jokes, his ever-growing repertoire of impressions (he did a spot-on Michele Ferrari: *Ahhhh, Tyler, you are too fat!*). I was the sidekick, the quiet, dry-humored one; the one who saw everything and didn't say much.

Lance was the big boss, lit up by this new life, by success. If he was intense before, now his intensity seemed to have doubled. Everything interested him; one day it would be tech stocks that were the *best fucking buy on the market*; the next it would be some bakery in Normandy that had the *best fucking bread you've ever tasted*; the next it would be about some band that was the *best fucking band you've ever heard*. The thing is, he usually was right.

Lance's eye was also on the competition. He spent a lot of time talking about Ullrich, Pantani, Zülle, and the rest. Lance knew a lot—who was working with which doctor, who was targeting which race, who was five kilos over-weight, who was getting divorced. Lance was like a one-man newspaper: you could go for a two-hour ride and get the scoop on the entire peloton.

Sometimes he was too talkative. I remember sitting at a restaurant on the Nice waterfront with him and Kevin, and Lance was talking about some new type of EPO he'd heard some Spanish riders were using. He was talking really loudly and openly, and not using any code words, and I got nervous, hoping there weren't any English-speakers in the next booth. I was so worried, in fact, I said something like "Hey, I think the walls might have ears." But he didn't seem to care. He kept right on talking. It was like his keeping EPO in his fridge. The rest of us were borderline paranoid about getting caught, while Lance acted like he was invulnerable. Or maybe acting in-vulnerable made him feel more secure.

While I learned a lot from Lance, my real education happened every few weeks, when Ferrari came to town. Ferrari was our trainer, our doctor, our god. Ferrari had a knack for designing sessions that were like torture devices: enough to almost kill us, but not quite. In later years we often heard Lance tell the public that Chris Carmichael was his official coach—and Carmichael built quite a business on that relationship. I know they were friends. But the truth is, during the years I trained with Lance, I don't recall Lance ever mentioning Chris's name or citing a piece of advice Chris had given him. By contrast, Lance mentioned Ferrari constantly, almost annoyingly so. *Michele says we should do this. Michele says we should do that.**

I had a lot to learn. Until then, I'd trained like most old-school bike racers trained—which is to say, by feel. Oh, I did intervals and counted hours, but I wasn't very scientific about it. You can see the proof in my daily journals, where most days are marked by a single number: how many hours I rode—the more, the better. That ended the second I set foot in Nice. Lance and Ferrari showed me there were more variables than I'd ever imagined, and they all mattered: wattages, cadence, intervals, zones, joules, lactic acid, and, of course, hematocrit. Each ride was a math problem: a precisely mapped set of numbers for us to hit—which makes it sound easy, but in reality it was incredibly difficult. It's one thing to go ride for six

---

* In his books and on his website, Carmichael asserts that he worked as Armstrong's coach throughout his seven Tour victories. In a *USA Today* interview in July 2004, Carmichael described a system in which Armstrong sent his daily training data to Ferrari, who forwarded them to Carmichael, who then adjusted Armstrong's training accordingly.

In interviews for *Lance Armstrong's War*, however, Ferrari said he had never communicated with Carmichael. "I do not work with Chris Carmichael," he said. "I work for Lance. Only Lance."

Here is what Postal riders say on the subject:

Jonathan Vaughters: "In two years, I never heard Lance refer to Chris one time."

Floyd Landis: "Give me a break. Carmichael's a nice guy, but he had nothing to do with Lance. Carmichael was a beard."

Christian Vande Velde: "Chris had nothing to do with Lance's daily training. I think his role was more like a friend, someone to talk about the bigger picture."

hours. It's another to ride for six hours following a program of wattages and cadences, especially when those wattages and cadences are set to push you to the ragged edge of your abilities. Supported by steady doses of Edgar and the red eggs, we trained like I'd never imagined was possible: day after day of returning home and falling unconscious into bed, utterly exhausted.

Every month or so, Ferrari would travel from his home in Ferrara and test us. His visits were like scientific experiments, only he was measuring the ways in which we were disappointing him. He always stayed at Lance and Kristin's, and so I'd wake up in the morning and ride over to see him. He'd be there with his scale, calipers, and blood spinner. Pinch pinch. Spin spin. He'd start to shake his head.

Aaaaaah, Tyler, you are too fat.

Aaaaaah, Tyler, your hematocrit is too low.

Ferrari liked to test us at the Col de la Madone, a steep twelve-kilometer climb just outside of Nice. Sometimes we would do a one-kilometer test, where we'd ride uphill repeatedly at gradually increasing wattages, and Ferrari would measure the lactate in our blood, charting the results on graph paper so we could figure out our thresholds (basically, how much power we could sustainably produce without burning out). Then, we'd ride the Madone full gas, revving our engines to the maximum. Riding well for Ferrari on the Madone felt almost as important as winning a race.

I tapped Ferrari for information; I used to write down questions on napkins so I'd remember to ask him. He taught me why hemoglobin was a better measure of potential than hematocrit, since hemoglobin comes closer to measuring oxygen-carrying capacity. He explained how a faster cadence put less stress on the muscles, transferring the load from the physical (the muscle fibers) to a better place: the cardiovascular engine and the blood. He explained that the best measure of ability was in watts per kilogram—the amount of power you produce, divided by your weight. He said that 6.7 watts per kilogram was the magic number, because that was what it took to win the Tour.

Michele was obsessed about weight—and I mean totally obsessed. He talked about weight more than he talked about wattage, more than he talked about hematocrit, which could be easily boosted with a little Edgar. The reason: losing weight was the hardest but most efficient way to increase the crucial watts per kilogram number, and thus to do well in the Tour. He spent far more time bugging us about diet than he ever did about our hematocrit. I remember laughing with Lance and Kevin about it: most people thought Ferrari was some crazed chemist, when to us he was more like a one-man Weight Watchers program.

Eating meals with Ferrari was a nightmare. He'd eagle-eye each bite that went into your mouth; a cookie or piece of cake would bring a raise of the eyebrow, and a disappointed look. He even persuaded Lance to buy a scale so he could weigh his food. I never went that far, but with his guidance, I tried different strategies: I drank gallons of sparkling water, trying to fool my stomach into thinking it was full. My body, which was being pushed like never before, didn't understand—it needed food, now! But here, as in so many things, Ferrari was right: as my weight dropped my performance improved. And kept improving.

This was a different sport than I was familiar with. Our opponents weren't other riders or the mountains or even ourselves; they were the numbers, these holy numbers that he put in front of us and dared us to chase. Ferrari turned our sport—a romantic sport where I used to climb on my bike and simply hope I had a good day—into something very different, something that was more like a chess game. I saw that the Tour de France wasn't decided by God or genes; it was decided by effort, by strategy. Whoever worked the hardest and the smartest was going to win.

This is probably a good time to address an important question: Was it possible to win a professional bike race clean during this era? Could a clean rider compete with riders on Edgar?

The answer is, depends on the race. For shorter races, even weeklong stage races, I think the answer is a qualified yes. I've won smaller four-day races paniagua with a hematocrit of 42. I've won time trials in similar condition. I've heard of other riders doing the same.

But once you get past a one-week race, it quickly becomes impossible for clean riders to compete with riders using Edgar, because Edgar is too big of an advantage. The longer the race, the bigger the advantage becomes—hence the power of Edgar in the Tour de France. The reason is cost, in the physiological sense. Big efforts—winning Alpine stages, winning time trials—cost too much energy; they cause the body to break down, hematocrit to drop, testosterone to dwindle. Without Edgar and the red eggs, those costs add up. With Edgar and the red eggs, you can recover, rebalance, and keep going at the same level. Dope is not really a magical boost as much as it is a way to control against declines.

That spring in Nice we trained harder and longer than I'd ever imagined I could train. It worked. Here are a couple of journal entries from 2000. (Note: By March 30, I had already been racing for nearly six weeks. Also, I wrote "HR" next to my hematocrit so that people would think it was my heart rate. Clever, eh?)

MARCH 30
Weight: 63.5 kg (139 pounds)
Body fat: 5.9 percent
Avg. watts: 371
Watts per kilo: 5.84
HR [hematocrit]: 43
Hemoglobin: 14.1
Max heart rate: 177
Madone time: 36.03

MAY 31
Weight: 60.8 kg (134 pounds)
Body fat: 3.8 percent
Avg. watts: 392
Watts per kilo: 6.45
HR [hematocrit]: 50
Hemoglobin: 16.4
Max heart rate: 191
Madone time: 32:32

In sixty days, I went from being in the middle of the pack to being within shouting distance of Ferrari's magic number for winning the Tour—a 10 percent improvement in a sport where half a percent can decide a big race. The timing was perfect for me, because the Dauphiné Libéré, the weeklong race in the French Alps that served as a traditional tuneup for Tour contenders, was just around the corner. I knew Lance wanted to win it, but I thought that perhaps I could acquit myself well, cement my role as his top lieutenant.

It was around this time that I started to notice a shift in my relationship with Lance. He knew my numbers. He saw where I was, and how fast I was improving. I noticed that on the times when we trained side by side, Lance would edge his front wheel ahead of mine. I'm stubborn, though, and I'd respond. It became a pattern: Lance would edge out six inches, and I would respond by putting my wheel one centimeter behind his. Then he'd edge out another six inches, and I'd respond—one centimeter behind. I always stayed one centimeter behind, to let him control the pace. That one centimeter separating us came to mean a lot. It was like a conversation, with Lance asking the questions.

How's that feel?
—Still here.
This?
—Still here.
Okay, this?
—Still here, dude.

At the time I was proud of it—of proving what a strong lieutenant I was. Only later did I realize how this contained the seeds of disaster.

★ ★ ★

The other part of my apprenticeship had to do with life at home. Haven's a natural organizer, and she dove into our new life in Nice. She took French lessons. She handled shopping, banking, paperwork, you name it. She found a great produce market and raided it every day; she would chop my salad into small bits, figuring it would take less energy to digest it. That was the kind of small but important touch that made me appreciate her. Haven wasn't just along for the ride, she was ready to do whatever it took to help me out, to be a part of our two-person team.

We got along great, with one exception. Walking. I know this sounds crazy, but one of the first rules I learned as I entered topflight bike racing was this: *If you're standing, sit down; if you're sitting, lie down; and avoid stairs like the plague.* Bike racing is the only sport in the world where the better you get, the more you resemble a feeble old man. I'm not sure of the physiology behind it, but the truth was, walking and standing for extended periods wore you out, made your joints ache, and thus set back your training. (Five-time Tour de France champion Bernard Hinault hated stairs so much that during some Tours, he would have his soigneurs carry him into the hotels rather than walk.) This meant that when Haven wondered if I wanted to go for a Sunday stroll on the beach, or a hike in the nearby mountains, or a walk to the corner market, I would usually beg off. *Sorry, hon, I gotta rest.*

I was kept busy, however, by other household errands, many of them revolving around Edgar. First I had to get it, which was more complicated now that the team was no longer carrying EPO to races. This meant buying the first of my many secret phones—prepaid cell phones. I'd use the secret phone to call del Moral or his assistant, Pepe Martí, and tell him I needed some "vitamins" or "allergy medication" or "iron tablets" or whatever code word we were using at the time. Then I'd drive to meet Pepe at some rendezvous point, and pick up a supply of red eggs and EPO from Dr. del Moral's clinic. I normally bought about twenty injections' worth, enough for about two months. I carried it in a soft-sided cooler with some ice packs, and del Moral would add a phony prescription for Haven—usually something about blood loss due to a menstrual condition—on the off chance I got stopped by the cops and searched, which, thank God, I never did.

Unlike Lance, I wasn't comfortable putting white boxes with the label AMGEN or EPREX next to my Diet Cokes. So I developed a system. First I soaked the outer cardboard packaging in water until it was unreadable, then I tore it up into tiny pieces and flushed it down the toilet. Then I used my thumbnail to peel the sticky labels off the glass EPO vials, which in that day were about an inch and a half tall and a half-inch wide, and flushed the labels as well. Then I wrapped the whole thing in tinfoil and put it in the back of the fridge, behind a pile of vegetables. Later, trying to be clever, I bought a fake root beer can with a secret screwtop compartment, like you'd order from the back of a comic book, but I worried someone would mistake it for a real can of root beer and try to drink it. Foil turned out to work best, because nobody wants to open up small, wrinkly packages that look like leftovers. The system worked well, except for one drawback: the balled-up labels were sticky, and tended to find their way into my shirt or pants pockets. Many times, I would be out at dinner or the grocery store, reach into my pocket to get something, and my hand would come out with an EPO label attached. Oops.

That was mostly it. No big menus of drugs; just Edgar and testosterone (Andriol). One red egg of Andriol every week or two during training was usually enough; though if you needed a smaller boost you could poke an egg with a safety pin, squeeze out some of the oil onto your tongue, and save the rest for later. Ferrari came up with a way of mixing Andriol with olive oil; he put it in a dark glass bottle with an eyedropper, for little boosts. I remember getting some of the oil from Lance at a race once: he held out the dropper and I opened my mouth like a baby bird. At del Moral's suggestion I tried some human growth hormone for one training bloc—a half-dozen injections over twenty days—but it made my legs feel heavy and bloated and made me feel like crap, so I stopped.

I took a shot of Edgar about every second or third day, usually 2,000 units, which sounds like a lot but in fact is only about the volume of a pencil eraser. I'd inject it under the skin, in either my arm or my belly; the needle was so small it barely left a mark. Quick-quick, and then you have a little sparkle in your blood.

When a vial was empty I'd wrap it in several layers of paper towel or toilet paper and pound it with a hammer or the heel of a dress shoe until the glass was crunched into tiny pieces. I'd take the broken-glass-and-paper-towel package to the sink and hold it under running water, removing all traces of EPO. Then I'd flush it all down the toilet or throw the wet mess in the garbage and cover it with the stinkiest stuff I could find: old banana peels, coffee grounds. I sometimes cut my hands on the glass, but overall it was a good system; I could sleep without being afraid of the French police raiding our house.

We could sleep, I mean. I didn't keep anything secret from Haven. She knew about the trips, the cost, my smash-and-rinse system, the whole thing. It would've felt wrong not to tell her, and besides, it was safer to keep both of us on the same page, on the off chance the police or a drug tester showed up. It wasn't like we chatted about EPO over toast and coffee. We both hated talking about it, hated dealing with it. But it was always there, floating in the air between us, that nagging, unpleasant chore we didn't like, but that had to be done. *No job too small or tough.*

I can't speak for everyone on the team, but it was my impression that most of the riders had the same full-disclosure policy when it came to their wives and girlfriends. There was only one notable exception: Frankie Andreu. Frankie was in a tougher spot because he was married to Betsy, and Betsy's attitude toward doping was the same as the pope's attitude toward the devil.

Betsy Andreu was an attractive, dark-haired Michigander with a big laugh and an open, no-bullshit manner that mirrored her husband's. She'd been in Lance's circle for years (Lance and Frankie had ridden for Motorola together from 1992 to 1996). Betsy's relationship with Lance had two chapters. In the first chapter, before cancer, Betsy and Lance had gotten along well.

They were both strong personalities who liked to argue about politics and religion (Lance was an atheist; Betsy was a practicing, pro-life Catholic). Lance trusted her to the point that he had Betsy vet his new girlfriends. (Betsy, who wasn't always so positive about the women Lance chose, had given an early thumbs-up to Kristin.) Lance trusted Betsy because with her, as with him, there were no gray areas. Betsy saw the world clearly—true and false, good and evil. They'd both hate to hear this, but they're more than a little bit alike.

Lance and Betsy's relationship had changed, however, one day in the fall of 1996, when a recently engaged Betsy and Frankie, along with a small group of friends, visited Lance's hospital room in Indianapolis as he was recovering from cancer. According to Betsy and Frankie, who later testified about the incident under oath, two doctors entered the room and began asking Lance a series of medical questions. Betsy said, "I think we should give Lance his privacy," and stood to leave. Lance urged them to stay. They did. Then Lance answered the questions. When the doctor asked if he'd ever used performance-enhancing drugs, Lance answered, in a matter-of-fact tone, yes. He'd used EPO, cortisone, testosterone, human growth hormone, and steroids. (Armstrong has testified under oath that this incident never happened.)

In my mind, this is a classic Lance moment, being cavalier about doping. This was the same urge that made Lance put his EPO in the front of his fridge in Nice and talk about it openly at a restaurant. He wants to minimize doping, show it's no big deal, show that he's bigger than any syringe or pill.

Inside that hospital room, Betsy and Frankie managed to keep their cool, but the second they stepped outside into the hallway, Betsy went ballistic. She told Frankie that if he was doing that shit, the wedding was off. Frankie swore to her he wasn't, and Betsy gradually calmed down. A few months later, they did get married, but Betsy never looked at Lance or the sport the same way again.

As you can imagine, this put Frankie in a tough spot, considering the demands of our profession. Lance and I often spoke openly about Ferrari and Edgar in front of our partners, but whenever Betsy was around, that changed. The phrase Frankie always used was *Betsy'll kill me*. He'd be particularly nervous before a group dinner. *Shut up about that stuff, guys—Betsy'll kill me.**

---

* After seeing Frankie's performance in the mountains of the 1999 Tour de France, Betsy confronted Frankie and asked him, "How the hell did you ride so well in the mountains?" Frankie refused to answer. Betsy drew her own conclusions: that Postal had a doping program, and that Ferrari and Armstrong were at the center of it.

In the years that followed, Betsy became a passionate anti-doping advocate, and a thorn in the side of Armstrong and Postal. Her involvement deepened in 2003 when she assisted David Walsh with his book *L.A. Confidentiel,* and when she was asked to testify under oath in 2005 about the 1996 hospital-room scene as part of Armstrong's legal battle with SCA Promotions. Over time, Betsy Andreu became a clearinghouse of information for journalists and anti-doping authorities alike.

"It's funny," she says of her role. "Lance likes to portray me as this fat, bitter, obsessed bitch who's out to get him. But all I've cared about from the beginning is to get the truth out."

Frankie, on the other hand, takes a different approach. While he gave a limited confession to *The New York Times* in 2006, in which he spoke of being introduced to performance-enhancing drugs in 1995 while on Motorola with Armstrong, and admitted to using EPO to prepare for the 1999 Tour de France, he mostly chooses to remain silent about doping—a stance

Frankie did what he had to do. Fortunately for him, it wasn't as much as Kevin, Lance, and I had to do. This was due to the fact that Frankie was a *rouleur*, a big guy, suited for grinding through flatter and rolling stages, and so required less Edgar and other therapy than we climbers did. If we had to tune our engines to 99 percent of capacity at the Tour, Frankie could gut it out while staying a little closer to *au naturale*.

While I admired Betsy's conscience, I didn't suffer any such hesitations myself. I was learning fast. With the help of Ferrari's spinner, I was learning to calibrate how much EPO I should take to fuel my increasingly intense training. Ferrari taught me that injecting EPO under the skin was like turning up the thermostat in a house: it worked slowly, causing your body to create more red blood cells over the next week or so. Add too little, and the house would be too cold—your hematocrit would be too low. Add too much, and the house would get too hot—you'd go over the 50 limit.

I got to where I could estimate my hematocrit level by the color of my blood. I'd stare at the little drops when Ferrari stuck my finger with a lancet when he gave a lactate test. If it was light and watery, my hematocrit was low. If it was dark, it was higher. I liked seeing that dark, rich color, all those cells crowding in there like a thick

that can create a unique tension in the small ranch home they share with their three children. In the summer of 2010, federal investigator Jeff Novitzky interviewed Frankie for two hours by phone. When Frankie hung up the phone, Betsy noticed he looked shaken. She asked him what he'd said. "I don't want to talk about it," Frankie said. Betsy phoned Novitzky and asked him. Novitzky laughed. "He's your husband," he said. "Go ask him."

soup, ready to go to work; it made me eager to train even harder.

Training felt like a game. How hard can you work? How smart can you be? How skinny can you get? Can you pit yourself against those numbers, and can you reach them? And then, behind all that, was always the anxiety that drove you, that kept you working: *Whatever you do, those other fuckers are doing more.*

The other game, however, had to do not with EPO, but with Lance—namely, how to get along with him. He's a touchy guy, and as the 2000 Tour grew closer, he got touchier. By June, the ragtag charm of the Bad News Bears seemed a million years old. Now he was tenser, more distant. He related to us less like a teammate than a CEO: hit your numbers, or else. Small things would set him off, and you knew it had happened when you got The Look—the long, unblinking three-second stare.

It's funny; the media would go on to treat The Look as if it were Lance's superpower, some-thing he unveiled at big moments in races, but to us, it was something that happened more often on the team bus or around the breakfast table. If you interrupted Lance while he was talking, you got The Look. If you contradicted what Lance was saying, you got The Look. If you were more than two minutes late for a ride, you got The Look. But the thing that really set off The Look was if you made fun of him. Underneath that tough exterior was an extraordinarily sensitive person. My teammate Christian Vande Velde once made fun of some new Nike shoes Lance was wearing one morning at breakfast. Christian is a great guy—he didn't mean anything by it, he was just trying to go with the flow, and gave Lance some frat-boy dig about his shoes. *Nice fucking shoes, dude!* Christian laughed. Lance got pissed, gave Christian The Look. And that was it. I'm sure that incident didn't end Christian's prospects on Postal. But it definitely didn't help.

But one of the biggest ways to piss off Lance was to complain about doping.

Jonathan Vaughters was probably the best example of this. With his probing mind, JV wasn't the kind of guy to accept doping at face value. He didn't just do whatever Lance and Johan said. He asked the questions nobody asked: Why are we doing this? Why doesn't the UCI enforce the rules? What's more, JV was twitchy when it came to the doping; he was always worried about police, or testers. He even talked about feeling guilty—and guilt was an emotion most of us had given up long ago. To Lance, JV's questions and doubts were proof that JV lacked the right attitude. I remember Lance bitching JV out after the 1999 Dauphiné when JV made the mistake of mentioning that he was happy finishing second in a stage—the position Lance liked to call "first loser." After the 1999 Tour, it was clear to everybody that JV didn't gel with Lance and Johan's system.

Vaughters left Postal in 2000 for the French team Crédit Agricole, where stricter French anti-doping laws kept the team in line. JV essentially curtailed his career in order to get away from the doping culture. But back then, Lance considered JV the king choad. To Lance's way of thinking, doping is a fact of life, like oxygen or gravity. You either do it—and do it to the absolute fullest—or you shut up and get out, period. No bitching, no crying, no splitting hairs. This made JV the worst kind of hyp-ocrite in Lance's eyes because he'd used his Postal results to sign a big two-year contract with Crédit Agricole, and therefore he owed it to his sponsor to get results—that's what they were paying him for. And suddenly JV was Mister Clean, moaning about doping, proclaiming his righteousness, finishing in the middle of the pack? Choad.*

Of course, there were more direct ways to cross Lance. One such incident happened in the spring of 2000 when we were finishing a six-hour training ride, climbing a narrow road toward my house. Lance and I were tired, dehydrated, hungry, ready to come home and take a nap. Then this small car comes tearing up the hill behind us at top speed, nearly hitting us, and the driver yells some-thing as he goes past. I'm mad, so I yell back at him. But Lance doesn't say anything. He just takes off, full speed, chasing the car. Lance knew the streets, so he took a short-cut and managed to catch the guy at the top, near a red light. By the time I got there Lance had pulled the guy out of his car and was pummeling him, and the guy was cowering and crying. I watched for a minute, not quite believing what I was seeing. Lance's face was beet red; he was in a full rage, really letting the guy have it. Finally, it was over. Lance pushed the guy to the ground and left him. We got back on our bikes and rode home in silence. In the days afterward Lance told that story to Frankie and

* Vaughters said that he had a candid conversation with Crédit Agricole's doctors before he signed the contract, in which he told them he'd been doping on Postal, and therefore couldn't be expected to achieve the same results. "It was all on the table before the contract was signed," he says.

Kevin as if it was funny, just another crazy-ass thing that happened in France. I tried to laugh along. But I couldn't. I kept picturing that guy on the ground, crying and pleading, and Lance pounding away. I'd seen more than I wanted to see.

This darker side of Lance stressed us out; but as far as the team's performance went, it served as fuel. He and Johan Bruyneel had Postal running like a Swiss watch. Better hotels. Better treatment from race organizers. Better planning. Better nutrition. Better sponsors. Better technology, including wind-tunnel testing. Our lives had the buzzy, connected feeling of being a part of something big and bold, like we were astronauts training for a NASA mission. Plus, there was the larger, simpler fact that we were riding our bikes together every day through some of the most beautiful terrain on the planet; the feeling of pushing yourself harder than you've ever pushed, making yourself into something powerful and new—and getting paid for it. On our rides, we'd sometimes catch each other's eye and smile, as if to say, can you believe how crazy this is?

As the 2000 Dauphiné Libéré approached, I was feeling quietly confident. I was lighter and stronger than I'd ever been. At my last fitness test, Ferrari had made a sound I'd never heard before—*Oooooh, Tyler!* The sound of approval.

I wanted to be strong, especially for the key day of the weeklong race, the stage on Mont Ventoux. There are lots of legendary climbs in France, but Ventoux might be the most legendary of all. It's called the Giant of

Provence, and it's tough enough that it has a body count: Tom Simpson, a British cyclist who died in 1967, over-dosing on a combination of exertion, brandy, and amphetamines.

For the first part of the Ventoux climb, I felt great. I should point out that when a bike racer says he feels great, he does not actually feel great. In fact, you feel like hell—you're suffering, your heart is jumping out of your chest, your leg muscles are screaming, flashes of pain are mov-ing around your body like so many strings of Christmas lights. What it means is that while you feel like crap, you also know the guys around you feel even crappier, and you can tell through their subtle expressions, the telltale signs, that they're going to crack before you do. Your pain, in that situation, feels meaningful. It can even feel great.

So here on Ventoux at the Dauphiné, I was feeling pretty great. Lance was next to me wearing the leader's yellow jersey, well positioned to clinch the overall. With 10 kilometers to go we were in the front group with an elite handful of contenders. My job was to cover the attacks—which meant to follow them, so no one got away. Once I did that, the plan was for Lance to bridge up and launch an attack of his own, and take the stage. It was straight out of Bike Racing 101: the old one-two.

The first part went well: I covered the attacks. I waited, expecting to see Lance riding across the gap.

No Lance.

I could hear Johan on the radio, urging him on. Time ticked by.

I started feeling a little nervous. I could see Alex Zülle

and Spanish climber Haimar Zubeldia catching up to me; others were following them. But where was Lance?

Time kept passing. Still more contenders rode up; it was getting crowded. But still no Lance. Then, Johan's voice.

Lance cannot make it. Tyler, you ride.

I checked with Lance.

Go. Just fucking go.

I launched an attack as we came along the Tom Simpson memorial, 1.5 kilometers from the lighthouse-like weather station that marks the top. I went deep, maybe deeper than I'd ever gone to that point. The world narrowed to a bright hallway. I felt Zülle and Zubeldia nearby, and then felt them fall away. I felt the spectators, felt my legs turning the pedals, but they didn't feel like my legs anymore. I gave everything; I made the last right switchback turn to the line, and crossed it.

Chaos. People grabbing me, screaming into my ear, media crowding around. I'm delirious.

I had won on Mont Ventoux.

A Postal soigneur grabbed me, wrapped a towel around my neck, and steered me toward the team bus. The bus was so quiet. I sat down, unclicked my helmet, let myself begin to take this in. It felt surreal.

I'd been stronger than all of them.

I was now a favorite to win the race.

The bus door wheezed open. Lance climbed grimly onto the bus, his head down. He sat ten feet away from me, toweled off, didn't say a word. I could see he was pissed. The silence became a bit uncomfortable.

A few seconds later the door opened again—Johan, a

concerned expression on his face, headed straight for Lance. He touched Lance on the shoulder, sat next to him, spoke softly, reassuringly. Like a nurse or a psychiatrist.

"This was no big deal, man," Johan said. "It was probably the altitude. Perhaps you have been training too hard, no? We will talk to Michele. The Tour doesn't even start for three weeks. Don't worry, there is plenty of time."

After a few minutes of this, Johan asked, "So, who won?"

Without looking up, Lance pointed at me.

Johan blushed, full red. He walked over and gave me an awkward hug, shook my hand, congratulated me. I think he felt embarrassed; he knew what a huge victory this was, and he'd ignored me completely. Now he made up for it.

But Lance stayed cranky. That night at dinner, when everybody was toasting my victory, he would barely make eye contact. It was like he was having an uncontrollable reaction, like an allergy: my success in the race—which was good for Postal, and therefore good for him—drove him bananas.

Late in the next day's stage, Lance and I managed to break away. I was thrilled at first—if we held on, it meant that I would go into the overall lead, and, just as important, we would show that Postal was the strongest team in the world going into the Tour. The thing was, it felt like Lance was trying to drop me. He kept accelerating on the final climbs, going way faster than we needed to go. Then he'd bomb the descents, going so fast we were both on the edge of crashing. I finally had to yell at him to slow down.

We crossed the line together. I finished that day wearing the leader's yellow jersey, the polka-dot jersey for best climber, the white jersey for most points. Winning the Dauphiné, a race whose former champions included Eddy Merckx, Greg LeMond, Bernard Hinault, and Miguel Indurain, instantly put me on the map. People started mentioning me as a possible Tour contender. But underneath, I was wondering about the way Lance had tried to break me on those climbs. It was the same pattern from our training rides: *Can you match this? This? This?*

The last night of the Dauphiné, Lance and Johan came to my hotel room. I expected them to talk about the race, or maybe plan for the upcoming Tour. Instead, they told me that on Tuesday, two days after the race ended, we were going to fly to Valencia to do a blood transfusion.

Chapter 7

THE NEXT LEVEL

AS A BIKE RACER, over time you develop the skill of keeping a poker face. No matter how extreme a sensation you feel—no matter how close you are to cracking—you do everything in your power to mask it. This matters in racing, when hiding your true condition from your opponents is a key to success, since it discourages them from attacking. Feel paralyzing pain? Look relaxed, even bored. Can't breathe? Close your mouth. About to die? Smile.

I've got a pretty good poker face; Lance has a great one. But there's one guy who's better than either of us: Johan Bruyneel. And it was never so well used as that night at the end of the 2000 Dauphiné, when he told me about the plans for the blood transfusion. I'd heard about transfusions before, but it was always theoretical and distant—as in, can you believe that some guys actually bank their blood, then put it back in before a race? It seemed weird, Frankenstein-ish, something for Iron Curtain

Olympic androids in the eighties. But Johan, when he explained the plan during the Dauphiné, made it sound normal, even boring. He's good at making the outrageous sound normal—it might be his greatest skill. It's something in his expression, in the certainty of his big Belgian voice, in the supremely casual way he shrugs while laying out the details of the plan. Whenever I watch the likable gangsters on *The Sopranos*, I think of Johan.

As Johan explained it, Lance, Kevin, and I would fly to Valencia. We would donate a bag of blood, which would be stored, and we'd fly home the next day. Then, at a key point during the Tour, we'd put the bag back in, and we'd get a boost. It would be like taking EPO, except better: there were rumors of an EPO test being developed for the 2000 Olympics, and word was, they might be using the test during the Tour. I listened to Johan, nodded, gave him my poker face. When I told Haven about it, she gave me the poker face right back (wives get good at it, too). But part of me was thinking, *What the hell?*

Maybe that's why I was late the Tuesday morning we left for Valencia. There was no reason to be late—everybody knew Lance despised lateness above all things—but on that crucial morning we were running late by a full ten minutes. I raced our little Fiat through the narrow streets of Villefranche; Haven was hanging on to the oh-shit bars, asking me to slow down. I kept speeding up. It was eight miles to the airport in Nice. During the trip, my cell phone rang three times. Lance.

Dude, where are you?

What's going on? We're about to take off.

How fast can that fucking car of yours go? Come on!

We screeched into the airport parking lot; I walked through the security area and onto the runway. I'd never been on a private jet before, so I took in the scene: the leather seats, the television, the little fridge, the steward asking me if I would like anything to drink. Lance acted casual, as if private jets were routine—which for him, they were. He'd been riding them fairly constantly since the previous July, courtesy of Nike, Oakley, Bristol-Myers Squibb, and the other corporations who were competing for the privilege of ferrying him around. The numbers were unbelievable. *USA Today* estimated Lance's income at $7.5 million, he was getting paid $100,000 per speech, and his new memoir, *It's Not About the Bike*, was an instant bestseller. You could feel the flow of money, the new possibilities it opened. Now we didn't have to drive to Valencia. We didn't have to worry about customs or airport security. The jet, like everything else, was now part of our tool box.

The engines revved, the wheels went up, and we were airborne. Below, we could see the Côte d'Azur, the mansions, the yachts; it felt surreal, like a fantasy world. In the plane, my lateness was forgiven. Lance was confident, happy, excited, and it was contagious. The confident feeling increased when we landed in Valencia and were met on the runway by the Postal team: Johan, Pepe Martí, and del Moral. They showed up with sandwiches, *bocadillos*—it was important to have a little something in our stomachs beforehand.

From the airport, we drove south for half an hour through a marshland as Johan and del Moral talked about the transfusion. It would be so simple, they said. So easy.

Extremely safe, nothing at all to worry about. I noticed Johan talked more to Kevin and me than to Lance, and that Lance didn't seem to pay attention; I got the feeling this wasn't Lance's first transfusion.

We pulled up near the village of Les Gavines at a beached whale of a hotel called the Sidi Saler, luxurious and quiet, free of the tourists who'd be arriving later in summer. We'd already been checked in; we took the elevator up to the fifth floor, moving through the deserted hallways. Kevin and I were directed into one room facing the parking lot; Lance got his own room next door.

I had expected to see a sophisticated medical setup, but this looked more like a junior-high science experiment: a blue soft-sided cooler, a few clear plastic IV bags, cotton balls, some clear tubing, and a sleek digital scale. Del Moral took over.

Lie on the bed, roll up your sleeve, give me your arm. Relax.

He tied a blue elastic band below my biceps, set an empty transfusion bag on a white towel on the floor next to the bed, and wiped the inside of my elbow with an alcohol swab. Then the needle. I'd seen a lot of needles, but this one was huge—about the size and shape of a coffee stirrer. It was attached to a syringe that was in turn attached to clear tubing that led to the waiting bag, with a small white thumbwheel to control flow. I looked away; felt the needle go in. When I looked again, my blood was pumping steadily into the bag on the floor.

You often hear "blood transfusion" tossed around in the same breath as "EPO" or "testosterone," as if it's all equivalent. Well, it's not. With the other stuff, you swallow a pill or put on a patch or get a tiny injection. But here you're watching a big clear plastic bag slowly fill up with your warm dark red blood. You never forget it.

I looked over to see Kevin hooked up in the same way. We could see our reflections on the closet-door mirror. We tried to cut the tension by comparing the speed with which our respective bags were filling: *Why are you going so slow? I'm dropping you, dude.* Johan shuttled between the rooms, checking on us, making small talk.

Every so often Pepe or del Moral would kneel down and take the bag in their hands, tilting it gently back and forth, mixing it with anticoagulant. They were gentle because, as they explained, the red blood cells were alive. If the blood was mishandled—shaken or heated, or left in a refrigerator beyond four weeks or so—the cells would die.

Filling the bags took about fifteen or twenty minutes. The bags plumped up until the scale showed we were done: one pint, 500 milliliters. Then, unhook: needle out. Cotton ball, pressure. Bags taped closed, labeled, and tucked into the blue cooler. Del Moral and Pepe headed out; they didn't say where, but we guessed it was to the clinic in Valencia and the refrigerator there, where the bags would be stored until we needed them three weeks later at the Tour.

I sat up, feeling woozy. Johan reassured us, soothed us: This feeling is normal. Take some B vitamins and an iron supplement. Eat a steak. Rest. Above all, do not take any EPO, because that will block your body's response of making more red blood cells. Your strength will come back soon.

Then we went on a ride south along the coast. We wore long sleeves to cover the Band-Aids on our arms, despite the afternoon heat. We weren't riding fast, but instantly we were breathing heavily, feeling light-headed. We reached a hill—a tiny pimple of a climb on the northern side of a town called Cullera. As we climbed, I felt worse and worse. We all started to gasp. We slowed to a pathetic crawl.

Just a few days ago, I'd been in the greatest shape of my life, beating some of the best athletes in the world on Mont Ventoux. Now I could barely make it up this tiny hill. We joked about it, because that was all we could do. But it was unnerving. It shook me deeply: my strength wasn't really in my muscles; it was inside my blood, in those bags.

The disconcerting feeling increased a couple days later, when Kevin and I rode the Route du Sud, a tough four-day race in southern France. When I arrived, my teammates were happy and impressed with my Dauphiné victory. Writers and the media were buzzing with expectation; other riders looked at me with new respect. After all, I had won on Ventoux; I was the next big thing, wasn't I?

In my depleted state, I was an utter embarrassment, a non-factor; Kevin wasn't any better. Instead of contending, I struggled to keep up with the pack. After the third stage, I was forced to do the one thing I hated most: abandon. I pulled off my race number, packed up my bags, and left the team hotel in shame.

When I returned to Nice, I expected Lance and Johan to apologize. After all, they were the ones who controlled the roster for the Route du Sud. In fact, Lance had originally been scheduled to be in the race, but he'd withdrawn at the last minute, citing his desire to rest before the Tour.

Lance or Johan could have made a phone call and taken Kevin and me off the Route du Sud team as well, spared us the humiliation and ensured our condition for the Tour. But they didn't. Neither Lance nor Johan ever said anything to me; they pretended our trip to Valencia hadn't happened. It was bullshit. That was a big learning experience for me—a teachable moment, as they say. I knew that protesting would do no good. I simply shut my mouth and did what I'd always done: keep going, no matter what. *No job too small or tough.*

Going into the 2000 Tour, Lance worried about two main problems. The first was that his physical margin over the rest of the field wasn't that big. As Lance pointed out, if you took out last year's early crash at the Passage du Gois, he had only beaten Zülle by 1:34 in the overall; and if Sestrière had been three kilometers longer, Zülle and the others would've caught him. The second factor was that the two big contenders who'd sat out the 1999 Tour would be back: Jan Ullrich and Marco Pantani.

Ullrich was like a superman—or, to be more accurate, a superboy. He'd come up training in East Germany, where the coaches lived by the maxim *Throw a dozen eggs against the wall, and keep the ones that don't break.* Ullrich was the unbreakable egg, a Cold War kid who, like Lance, had grown up without a father and, with the help of the East German state, had turned his energy into the single most impressive physique in cycling history. Ullrich's body was unlike any other rider's I'd ever seen. I'd sometimes try to ride next to him just so I could watch: you could actually see the muscle fibers moving. He was the only rider I've ever seen whose veins were visible under the Lycra. His mind wasn't bad, either: Ullrich had a remarkable ability to push himself, to go deep. In the 1997 Tour, when he was only twenty-three, I'd watched Ullrich win the hardest stage I've ever ridden, 242 kilometers over eight hours through the Pyrenees; he even destroyed the mighty Riis. Despite that imposing physique, Ullrich was a gentle soul, a nice guy who had a friendly word for everyone. His weakness was discipline—he struggled with his weight—but he had the ability to rise to the occasion and deliver a monster ride when you least expected it.

If Ullrich was a superboy, Pantani was more of a mystic: a small, shy, dark-eyed Italian who, when on form, was the best climber in the world. Pantani was a mix of artist and assassin: vain enough to get cosmetic surgery to pin back his prominent ears, tough enough to be able to win races in the worst conditions. He'd defeated Ullrich in the 1998 Tour, outriding "Der Kaiser" through a freezing storm to Les Deux Alpes. Since getting popped for high hematocrit the previous year, Pantani had struggled. He'd wrecked two sports cars and written open letters to his public that spoke of "a difficult period with too many inner problems." Still, Pantani would be out to reclaim his title, and with his climbing ability, he was dangerous. If Lance cracked in the mountains, Pantani could make him pay.

Lance talked about them constantly. Ullrich and Pantani; Pantani and Ullrich. He tracked their training, trawling the Internet for articles from obscure newspapers in Frankfurt and Milan. For a while Lance had so much information I thought he had someone working for him—I pictured a young intern in a cubicle somewhere, compiling reports. But after a while I realized it was all Lance. He needed to gather the information so he could convert it into motivational fuel. If Ullrich was in good shape, that motivated Lance to train harder. If Ullrich was overweight (as was the case that spring), then that also motivated Lance to train harder, to show Der Kaiser who was boss.

The 2000 Tour was really more like a series of boxing matches. Lance vs. Ullrich was over pretty quickly. First Lance beat Ullrich decisively in the prologue. Then he spent a few flat stages getting under Ullrich's skin. There are a thousand ways to intimidate someone in a bike race, and Lance knew every one of them. To chat when things are tough. To take a bite of food or a long drink when you're going fast, to show that you can. To accelerate quickly; to ride forward along the outside of the peloton, against the wind, with ease. He showed Ullrich over and over who was stronger. And Ullrich had no answer for any of it. By the first climb to the Spanish ski town of Hautacam, Lance had Ullrich in his pocket.

Lance vs. Pantani, though, was another matter entirely. Pantani was impetuous, romantic, the kind of person who in a slightly different life would have been a bullfighter or an opera star. He wouldn't rest until he'd made an impact on the race. Lance wanted things to be logical, and

Pantani wasn't logical, and Lance hated it. Even though Pantani was behind by a handful of minutes, we all knew that he would attack Lance on stage 12 on Mont Ventoux, where Lance had suffered during the Dauphiné. This suited Pantani's love of drama; it also suited us, because it was where Lance and Johan had planned to make our chess move.

After stage 11 finished, we traveled to a postcard of a town near Ventoux called Saint-Paul-Trois-Châteaux, where we'd spend the rest day before stage 12. We stayed at Hôtel l'Esplan, which was great not just because the owner gave the entire hotel to our team, or because they had a nice dining room, but also because some of the rooms were arranged as suites. They gave Kevin, Lance, and me one such pair of rooms that shared an arched entry; Kevin and I roomed together, as usual, and Lance was across the small foyer.

That night, before dinner, we did the transfusion in our rooms. The bags of our blood were taped to the walls above our beds with thick swatches of white athletic tape. The bags were shiny, swollen like berries. Johan went to the doorway, standing guard against any passersby. Kevin and I lay down like mirror images; through the open door, I could see Lance's sock feet, his arm, the tubing.

Del Moral and Pepe were fast and efficient: the blue rubber band to make the vein protrude, the needle pointing toward the heart, the wheel control to make the blood flow. They opened the valve and I watched my blood run down the tube, through the needle, and into my arm, and felt a chill. Goosebumps. Del Moral noticed, and explained that the blood had recently come out of the cooler; they kept it on ice to lower the risk of infection.

The transfusion took about fifteen minutes. We distracted ourselves by kidding around, talking trash, our voices echoing through the open door—*We're gonna throttle those guys on Ventoux*. Maybe we talked that way to reassure ourselves that this strange process was okay (because after all, they were all doing the same thing, right?), maybe to cover up any lingering feelings of guilt.

From the archway, Johan looked on approvingly. I watched my blood bag slowly empty, the last drops flow down the tube; del Moral cut it off just as the last red blood cells went in. I never asked what happened with the empty bags; I assumed del Moral and Pepe carried them to some anonymous dumpster miles away; more likely they cut them into tiny pieces and flushed them down the hotel toilet. We headed down to dinner. Everybody else was in shorts and short sleeves. The three of us, still chilled, kept our sweatsuits on.

At dinner, I noticed a strange sensation: I felt good. Normally at this point in the Tour, you feel a bit like a zombie—tired, shuffling, staring. Now, however, I felt springy, healthy. Euphoric, even, as if I'd had a couple cups of really good coffee. I caught sight of myself in a mirror: I had some color in my cheeks. Lance and Kevin seemed energized too. We relaxed through the rest day, went on a ride, got ready.

Writers like to get poetic about Ventoux. They say it's a moonscape of white rock, a windswept wasteland, an "alabaster death-head," blah blah. When you race it, however, you're reading a different kind of story: the faces and body language of the riders around you. You're looking for a tight grip on the handlebars. A hesitation or stiffness in the pedal stroke. Bobbing shoulders. A glance downward at the legs, puffy eyes, a gaping mouth, anything that suggests an impending crack. As we started toward Ventoux, I expected to see a lot of guys falling away around me.

The plan was to have Kevin and me go as hard as we could from the bottom of the climb, to burn off most of the contenders and let Lance save his strength as long as possible. When the race reached the pine forest at the foot of Ventoux, we revved—first me, then Kevin. Sure enough, the race blew apart and was soon down to a dozen or so riders; Johan was yelling into the radio that this was good, good, good. But strangely enough, I didn't feel all that great. My legs were thick, waterlogged. I pushed hard, bumped against that old, familiar wall sooner than I'd expected. I pushed harder, but couldn't seem to get past it. I began to slow. I felt weird, a little out of sorts—maybe my transfusion hadn't worked like it was supposed to, maybe my body hadn't reacted properly.

It would take me a couple of years to figure this out, but I hadn't yet learned how my body reacted to a transfusion. When you have more RBCs, your body doesn't obey the same rules: you can go harder than you think you can. Your body might be screaming in the same old way, but you can push through if you ignore all those signals and just ride. Later, I'd learn how to do that.

As I was slowing down, Pantani was coming back. Say what you will about his sometimes overdramatic personality, underneath he was one tough son of a bitch. Pantani somehow hauled himself back to the lead group and then, inconceivably, he was attacking, riding off the front. Lance let Pantani run a few hundred yards ahead, then counterattacked. Even now, when I watch it on video, I can't quite believe the speed Lance was traveling; the way he gobbles up the distance, sprinting up Ventoux like he's sprinting for a city-limits sign on a training ride. He caught up to Pantani and they rode together through the white rock, with Lance all the while showing Pantani how much stronger he was. Pantani could only follow, hanging on with his fingernails. It was spectacular. "They rode like the damned" was how fellow contender José Jiménez put it. By the time they reached the top, Lance had proved he was the strongest, so definitively that he eased off and let Pantani take the stage victory.

That moment should have ended the battle: Lance by TKO. But that didn't happen. Pantani got pissed off that Armstrong had gifted him Ventoux (the Italian didn't want any charity), and decided to make our lives hell. For the next few days he attacked, over and over. Crazy, hopeless, romantic attacks, fueled by his own pride and who knows what else. This created a cascade of problems, because Kevin and I couldn't keep up with Pantani, and a small group of Spanish riders—most notably a couple of tiny, tireless climbers named Roberto Heras and Joseba Beloki—could. This left Lance spending too much of the race isolated, alone, without teammates for support for much of the stages.

The worst came on stage 16, from Courchevel to Morzine, when Pantani took off alone early in the race, a suicide move we figured would soon end. But it didn't end. Pantani kept driving the pace; he didn't slow down;

in fact, he kept speeding up. We chased as hard as we could, but we weren't reeling him in. There was only one thing to do: Lance told Johan to get Ferrari on the phone.

The conversation was brief—I could picture Ferrari with his graph paper, running the numbers—and the answer came back: the pace was too fast. Pantani would crack. He could not keep this up. And Ferrari was right, as always. On the last climb, a nasty 12-kilometer ascent called the Joux Plane, Pantani finally cracked.

The problem was that Lance cracked too. Early in the climb, while he was alone, Lance started to slow. He tried to hide it for a while, but soon it was obvious: his face went white, his shoulders started rolling, and soon Ullrich was riding up the road, his superman legs churning as he left Lance in the dust. This was Ullrich's big chance, and Lance's nightmare. For the next twenty minutes, they both rode to their limits—Ullrich sprinting, Lance following more stiffly, more frantically, his expression frozen in exhaustion and fear. Lance showed a lot of toughness that day; he lost only one and a half minutes, when he could have easily lost ten.

After stage 16, Lance looked terrible: pale, squinty, puffy eyes, with dark circles underneath. In interviews, he called Pantani "a little shit-starter," which was true enough; the problem was that Postal didn't have any shit-stoppers—nobody strong enough to ride Pantani down.

Luckily for Lance and us, Pantani had used up all his ammunition, and abandoned the race the next day, citing illness. Lance recovered, and we made it to Paris without any problems to win his second Tour. We did the celebration at the Musée d'Orsay again, but underneath the triumph there was a note of concern. Pantani, single-handed, had nearly derailed Lance's victory. We were lucky Ullrich hadn't brought his A game, lucky that Pantani had eventually cracked, lucky that Lance had only lost a couple minutes on the Joux Plane. And Lance and Johan weren't the kind to rely on luck.

That's when the rumors started that Postal was going to sign more high-profile climbers. The obvious candidate was Roberto Heras, the Pantani-size Spaniard who'd finished fifth in the 2000 Tour and who'd go on to win the Tour of Spain that fall. But he seemed a long shot for obvious reasons: his existing contract with Kelme contained a $1 million buyout fee (more than Kevin and I made together) and our entire team budget was $10 million. We didn't seem to have the space to sign such an expensive rider, so I disregarded the rumors. I thought Postal's lineup was solid, and would stay together for years to come. In retrospect, I should have seen it coming.

A few weeks after the Tour, Lance and I were training together near Nice, and he started talking about Kevin. Lance was not happy. He said Kevin had approached Johan asking for more money—a two-year deal, with a significant bump in salary. Lance shook his head.

"I don't know who the fuck Kevin thinks he is," he said.

I remember being a little confused, thinking to myself that this was Kevin Frigging Livingston, the guy who had just helped Lance win two Tours in a row, who had sacrificed his place in the overall standings to support Lance, who had visited Lance in the hospital when he had cancer, who had been his closest friend. But to Lance, that wasn't the question. Kevin was good, but Kevin's performance was replaceable. Therefore, Kevin was replaceable.

"Kevin thinks he's gonna get paid," Lance said. "Well, he's not gonna get shit."

A few weeks later, I was riding with Lance, and he started talking about Frankie Andreu. Apparently Frankie had also asked for a raise, and Lance was not happy about that either.

"Frankie thinks he's gonna get paid. Well, he's not gonna get shit."[*]

It wasn't personal, it was mathematical. If Lance could gain a few seconds by making a helmet lighter, he made it happen. If Lance could save time by using a private jet, he made it happen. If Lance could free up salary money by cutting a couple of old friends from the team, he made it happen.

Neither Livingston nor Andreu was offered a contract for 2001. Kevin wound up on Telekom, riding for Jan Ullrich (in the press, Lance was unmerciful, comparing it to American general Norman Schwarzkopf going to work for Communist China), and Frankie simply retired. I think he was heartbroken; he'd ridden with Lance almost his entire career, and he didn't want to start over with another team. Their salary money was spent on signing the Spanish duo of Heras and his Kelme teammate

---

[*] Betsy Andreu says that Armstrong told Frankie that it was Thom Weisel's decision. "Lance said, 'It's not me; I want you on the team; it's Thom who's cutting the budget.' Even though it didn't make any sense—I mean, how could they be cutting the budget when they've just won two Tours?—Frankie believed Lance, and that was a mistake."

Chechu Rubiera, and the Colombian Victor Hugo Peña of Vitalicio Seguros, a trio who quickly became known as the Spanish Armada. Just like that, the Bad News Bears were gone.

The trolls showed up that fall as well. A French TV station had followed del Moral and Postal chiropractor Jeff Spencer during the 2000 Tour and filmed them disposing of syringes, bloodied compresses, and a drug called Actovegin. The French were making a big deal out of it, launching an official police investigation into the matter.

We had, in fact, used Actovegin, not only in 2000 but also in 1999. It was an injection del Moral gave some of the team just before a handful of big Tour stages, in order to increase oxygen transport, and which was undetectable in doping tests. But Postal handled this scandal with growing skill. First, they came up with some plausible medical reason for the team to have been carrying the substance (they said head mechanic Julien DeVriese was diabetic, and that it was also used for healing skin abrasions from road rash). Then they framed the story as if they were the victims of some unfair tabloid journalism setup. In addition, Lance scored style points by referring to the drug in the media as "Activo-something," as if he hadn't the foggiest idea how to pronounce it. The investigation came to nothing, and was eventually dropped. But it had one major effect: it got Lance out of France for good. In October he phoned me, saying that he had had enough of the fucking French. He was selling his place in Nice, getting out, now. I should, too. Where should we move?

I wasn't happy about leaving France; Haven and I

loved living in Villefranche—the community, the training, the friendships. But Lance was the boss. Kevin and
Frankie weren't on the team anymore. Life was moving
on.

I told Lance about Girona, that ancient walled Spanish
city I'd lived in before coming to France. I told him about
its cool restaurants, its decent training nearby, the half-
dozen other American riders who lived there, including
several of our teammates. As an additional plus, we all
knew the Spaniards were far less strict about doping; no
gendarmes raiding hotel rooms, no dumpster-diving
reporters. The decision took five minutes. We were
headed to Girona.

Chapter 8

LIFE IN THE NEIGHBORHOOD

DURING MY CAREER, JOURNALISTS often used the term "arms race" to describe the relationship between the drug testers and the athletes, but that wasn't quite right, because it implied that the testers had a chance of winning. For us, it wasn't like a race at all. It was more like a big game of hide-and-seek played in a forest that has lots of good places to hide, and lots of rules that favor the hiders.

So here's how we beat the testers:

- Tip 1: Wear a watch.
- Tip 2: Keep your cell phone handy.
- Tip 3: Know your glowtime: how long you'll test positive after you take the substance.

What you'll notice is that none of these things are particularly difficult to do. That's because the tests were very easy to beat. In fact, they weren't drug tests. They were more like discipline tests, IQ tests. If you were careful and paid attention, you could dope and be 99 percent certain that you would not get caught.

Early in my career (from 1997 to 2000) the testers were easy to deal with because they mostly didn't exist. You got tested at races only, and then only if you won a stage or were unlucky enough to have your name be among the one or two names drawn for the occasional random test. So all you had to do was to follow the team doctor's instructions and make sure you stopped using a certain number of days before the race. Remember, until 2000 there was no test for EPO, only the 50 percent hematocrit limit to worry about, and that was simple to manage with spinners and experience. Glowtime for the red eggs was three days, so that's basically all I had to worry about.

Around 2000, very slowly, out-of-competition testers started showing up. I volunteered for the inaugural testing program of the U.S. Anti-Doping Agency (USADA) because I wanted to ride in the Olympics, and I thought declining to volunteer might arouse suspicion. Testing was quarterly, to establish baseline values, with only a tiny handful of out-of-competition tests. Still, we had to make adjustments. One time, before the 2000 season, I asked Lance to overnight me some EPO from Austin to Marblehead so my blood values for the quarterly test would be more consistent. (I figured that having your hematocrit leap from 39 to 49 might draw attention.)

USADA called them "surprise" drug tests, but they usually weren't all that surprising. In Girona, we had a built-in advantage because the testing organization would send one person to test all the Girona cyclists. Whoever got tested first immediately phoned his friends to tell them (see Tip 2); word got around fast. So if you happened to be glowing, you could take evasive measures.

Ducking the out-of-competition tests was fairly easy. The testing agencies use what is known as a whereabouts program: you were supposed to inform them of your location at all times, and if you failed to do so, you could be penalized—given a strike. Three strikes in an eighteen-month period was supposed to lead to a sanction, in theory—but that rule had never been tested in court. One trick was to be vague in the whereabouts forms (I used to write "roadways, eastern MA, southern NH, 100 mile radius from Marblehead, MA"). Another trick was to change your plans at the last minute, so they were never quite sure where you were. The last trick was that when the tester showed up and you thought you might be glowing, you didn't answer the door.

The nightmare scenario was if the tester snuck up on you at the wrong time. Stories were around: One rider got busted when a tester hid in a parking garage and surprised him. I heard that one Tour contender had installed a set of mirrors near the doorway of his house so he could secretly observe who was coming. It sounds like paranoia, but from our point of view, it was merely being practical. I considered adding a back door to my Girona apartment so I could come and go more inconspicuously, and tried to minimize my time outside my front door, where a tester might waylay me unexpectedly. Whenever I returned from a training ride, I always came from the uphill side, zooming down the street, sunglasses on. I kept my house key in my right hand, the quicker to use it. I treated our Girona apartment like the Bat Cave—once I was inside, with the door locked behind me, I was safe.

Riders who lived with girlfriends or wives had a big advantage: a live-in scout who could deflect the testers, or cover for them. Haven and I developed a shorthand. If the doorbell rang unexpectedly, she'd lock eyes with me and ask, "You're good?" My answer was almost always yes, I'm good.

In late 2000, shortly after Haven and I bought a house in Marblehead, the doorbell rang. Haven did the check-in, and this time I shook my head. I wasn't good. In fact, I was glowing—I'd recently taken some testosterone (my personal doctor said mine was low, and it was prescribed, but still, I might have tested positive).

"Mister Hamilton? I'm here from USADA to administer a doping test."

Haven and I looked at each other for a long second. Then, moving as one, we hit the deck—we lay flat on our bellies on the tile floor of our new kitchen.

"Hello? Anybody there?"

We crawled across the floor and into the safety of the living room, and listened to the knocking. We put them off for the day. I fudged my whereabouts form, drank a ton of water, peed a lot. Then, when I was sure I wasn't glowing, I took the test.

Another way to hide was through the use of TUEs—therapeutic use exemptions, which were mostly used for cortisone. The UCI permits riders to use certain substances with a doctor's prescription. So the team doctors would invent some phantom problem—a bad knee, a saddle sore—and write a note allowing you to use cortisone or some similar substance. The only trick to it was remembering what made-up ailment the doctor had given you—was it your right knee that was supposed to be injured, or your left knee? Before races, I'd sometimes check the paperwork to make sure I knew which knee to complain about if the testers happened to ask.

The best way to hide, though, was simply by reducing glowtime to a minimum. Because the best, most liberating rule of drug testing is this: the testers can only visit you between 7 a.m. and 10 p.m.* This means that you can take anything you like, as long as it leaves your system in nine hours or less. This makes 10:01 p.m. a particularly busy time in the world of bike racers. If you're in Spain, you're twice lucky, because given the nocturnal Spanish customs (dinner often starts at 10:30 p.m.), the testers almost never turn up at 7 a.m.; it's more like noon, or later. (One tester, a considerate older gentleman who lived an hour away in Barcelona, used to telephone the night before to make

* According to the code of the World Anti-Doping Agency, athletes were required to make themselves available for testing twenty-four hours a day. In practice, however, testers seem to have obeyed the 7 a.m.–10 p.m. window. In fact, French law decrees that any testing organization, national or international, must schedule tests between 6 a.m. and 9 p.m.; Spain passed a similar law in 2009. The reasoning was (1) to protect athletes' privacy; (2) the mistaken belief that any drug that was in an athlete's body at bedtime would still be detectable in the morning.

Bernhard Kohl, an Austrian cyclist who finished third in the 2008 Tour de France before being suspended for a blood booster and stripped of the result, told *The New York Times*, "I was tested 200 times during my career, and 100 times I had drugs in my body. I was caught, but 99 other times, I wasn't. Riders think they can get away with doping because most of the time they do."

sure we were in town, so he didn't waste a trip.) But the best way to reduce glowtime was to have a smart doctor who could find new ways of administering drugs so they left your body more quickly, but still had the desired effect. And when it came to doctors, we had the smartest: Ferrari.

The test for EPO is a good example of how big an advantage Ferrari was to us. It took the drug-testing authorities several years and millions of dollars to develop a test to detect EPO in urine and blood. It took Ferrari about five minutes to figure out how to evade it. His solution was dazzlingly simple: instead of injecting EPO subcutaneously (which caused it to be released over a long period of time), we should inject smaller doses directly into the vein, straight into the bloodstream, where it would still boost our red blood cell counts, but leave our body quickly enough to evade detection. Our regimen changed. Instead of injecting 2,000 units of Edgar every third or fourth night, we injected 400 or 500 units every night. Glowtime minimized; problem solved. We called it microdosing.*

The trick with getting Edgar in your vein, of course, is that you have to get it in the vein. Miss the vein—inject it in the surrounding tissue—and Edgar stays in your body far longer; you might test positive. Thus, microdosing requires a steady hand and a good sense of feel, and a lot of practice; you have to sense the tip of the needle

---

* This proved to be a good example of the information gap between testers and athletes. Dr. Michael Ashenden, the hematologist who helped develop the EPO and transfusion tests, was not aware of the in-the-vein microdosing strategy until Floyd Landis explained it to him in 2010.

piercing the wall of the vein, and draw back the plunger to get a little bit of blood so you know you're in. In this, as in other things, Lance was blessed: he had veins like water mains. Mine were small, which was a recurring headache. If you miss the vein you can see the EPO forming a small bubble beneath the skin. I've seen that start to happen a few times; fortunately for me, I stopped it in time, and was lucky not to be tested the following day. A few millimeters one way or the other can end a career. Sometimes, when riders unexpectedly test positive, I wonder if that's the reason.

Of course, EPO wasn't the only thing that could be microdosed: testosterone worked that way, too. Around 2001 the red eggs were used less than testosterone patches, which were more convenient. They were like big Band-Aids with a clear gel in the center; you could leave one on for a couple of hours, get a boost of testosterone, and by morning be clean as a newborn baby.

Still, we had to be careful. One of my closer calls happened while I was living in Girona. We had some houseguests visiting, an old high school friend and his wife, and perhaps because I was distracted, I left my testosterone patch on for too long—for six hours instead of two hours. When I realized it—when I felt the crinkle of the patch on my stomach—I had a sinking feeling. Now I was glowing, and would be for about a day.

I went for a ride early the following morning, and as luck would have it, the testers showed up while I was out. Haven called me, and so instead of going home, I rode to a hotel and spent the night—which made for some awkwardness around our houseguests, but ended up being the right thing to do. Taking a strike wasn't a big deal. Getting caught, testing positive, would have been a catastrophe: I'd lose my job, my sponsors, my team, and my good reputation. I'd jeopardize Postal, and the jobs of my friends. Due to the French investigation, our 2001 Postal contracts contained a clause that allowed Postal to terminate the contract of any rider who violated anti-doping rules. Like Lance and everybody else, I lived my life one slip-up, one glowing molecule, away from ruin and shame.

Compared to the cluelessness of the testers, Lance's senses were dialed in tight, particularly when it came to doping. He watched everyone; he looked for strange leaps in performance; he paid attention to who was working with which doctor. He wanted to sort out who was doping more, being aggressive, ambitious, innovative—in short, who needed to be watched.

Leading up to the 2001 Tour, Lance's radar was working overtime. He knew that Ullrich was training in South Africa—and was it a coincidence that a blood substitute called Hemopure had just been approved over there? He knew that a lot of the up-and-coming Spanish riders were working with a Madrid doctor named Eufemiano Fuentes. He knew that Pantani was falling off the deep end, getting into cocaine and other recreational drugs. Above all, he knew that the new EPO test was going to be introduced in the spring, and that there were new, un-detectable forms of EPO being developed. The game was constantly changing.

To stay ahead, Lance would use races for gathering

information, digging for gossip, getting some inside knowledge. Lance would pull alongside someone—often the Italians or the Spanish, who were known for being chatty—and simply ask them, in that straightforward, irresistible Lance way, What was going on, what was new? Who was flying? How did Ullrich look? How was Pantani climbing? What doctor were they working with? Riders were eager to get on Lance's good side; they knew he had the power to help or hurt them.

Lance had information on me, too. One day while we were riding in the hills above Nice, he mentioned that Postal's budget was being stretched because of the expensive new signings of Heras and the Armada. Then he mentioned something he should not have known: the $100,000 contractual bonus I'd just earned for being part of the Tour-winning team.

I was unnerved—my personal contract with Postal was nobody's business, especially not Lance's. Then I was more unnerved, because Lance asked if I would forgo my $25,000 Tour bonus from him and give it to the team, to ease the budget strain. He floated it like it was a cool, innovative idea; and with the implication that, if I was a team player, I'd agree.

In retrospect, his idea looks wrong on a bunch of levels—a violation of my privacy, not to mention of common sense: Lance could easily afford to pay me the money I was due; he earned four times that for a one-hour speech. But at the time, I didn't see much choice other than to say, Yes, sure, boss, I'll chip in. I'd seen what happened with Kevin and Frankie. I knew fighting with Lance was a no-win proposition.

In early 2001, a few of us on the A team held an early season training camp in Tenerife, in the Canary Islands off the coast of Africa. It was one of Lance's MacGyver deals—a phone call, a private-jet ride, a sense of secrecy, even from the rest of the team—it was just going to be Lance, myself, the three new Spanish guys, Johan, Ferrari, and a couple of soigneurs.

To call Tenerife remote is putting it nicely—the islands are dusty red rocks, the place they used to film movies like *Journey to the Center of the Earth*. We stayed in a big empty hotel on the top of a volcano; I roomed with Roberto Heras, and for almost two weeks we did nothing but ride, sleep, and eat. Ferrari brought his daughter along, a skinny, dark-haired teenager who looked like a mini Michele. I remember sitting at the dinner table, with two Ferraris eyeballing us, watching everything we ate.

Lance was watching too. He tended to treat us like we were extensions of his body, especially when it came to eating. Guys on the team still told the story about the time a couple of years earlier in Belgium when Lance had indulged himself by eating a piece of chocolate cake during a training camp. It must've been pretty good cake, because then Lance ate another piece. Then, unthinkably, he ate a third. The other Postal riders watched him eat with a sinking feeling: they knew what was going to happen. The next day in training was supposed to be an easy day. But the cake changed that. Instead, Lance had the team do a brutal five-hour ride, to burn off the cake only he had eaten. When he sinned, the whole team had to pay the price.

The Armada turned out to be nice guys: Chechu

Rubiera was a true gentleman and a former law student; Victor Hugo Peña was a strapping Colombian with a shark tattoo on his left shoulder and an iron work ethic; Roberto Heras was a quiet, boyish guy who barely said three words. One night on Tenerife Roberto finally spoke a complete sentence.

He asked, "How does a cyclist put sugar in his coffee?"

We shook our heads. Roberto picked up the sugar packet and flicked it with his finger, like he was flicking a syringe. Everybody cracked up.

We rode for five to seven hours each day through this red moonscape. Each night we returned to the empty hotel (it was the tourist off-season). It felt like being in *The Shining*. We ate in the empty dining room. We wandered the halls. Roberto would try to say, "I am so fucking bored." But since his English wasn't great, he would say, "I am so fucking boring." That became our motto for the trip. *I am so fucking boring.*

But it wasn't all boring. Michele was giving microdoses of EPO every couple of days, usually in the evenings. This meant we had to be on our toes, in case a tester decided to show up (we knew this was highly unlikely, given the distance and expense, but still). One afternoon, Lance spotted an unfamiliar man in the hotel lobby and the guy didn't look like a tourist. He was asking questions, looking around. Lance sprinted for the hotel's back door. It turned out the man was a reporter from a Tenerife newspaper who'd heard we were staying there and was merely hoping for an interview.

We returned from Tenerife exhausted but ready for the season. My spring races went well. Then, in April, I had a small disaster: I crashed at Liège–Bastogne–Liège and broke my elbow. I wish it had been something dramatic, but it was a typical stupid crash: the guy in front of me went down, and I plowed into him. One second, I was on track for a good spring; the next, I was in a splint. I decided to return to Marblehead for a few weeks to recuperate; the plan was, I'd return in mid-May for Tour training camps and for my big opportunity of the season, the Tour of Switzerland. I was psyched for Switzerland, because Johan had told me that I would be the team leader for that race—a huge opportunity, and a big responsibility. I brought a few vials of Edgar in my luggage. In Marblehead, I trained as if I were alongside Lance; I ate as if Ferrari were watching me. I used plenty of Edgar (I didn't have a spinner, so I was operating by feel). I saw my mom and dad and brother and sister, but not as often as I would have liked. I concentrated on my training. I was aiming at the Tour of Switzerland like a laser beam, determined not to let this injury set me back.

When I returned to Europe in May, I was in good shape. Very good shape, in fact. I went straight to Dr. Ferrari at his home in Ferrara. He did his usual assessments—body fat, hematocrit, weight—and he smiled. Then we did a fitness test on the Monzuno climb, which was one of Ferrari's favorites: a four-kilometer climb that rises 1,250 feet at a 9 percent grade through farms and olive trees. Lots of great riders had tested themselves there; in fact, Lance held the Monzuno record. At least until that day. When I got to the top, Ferrari was smiling like I'd never seen him smile. I'd broken Lance's record. Smashed it, in fact.

That was a good feeling.

The feeling multiplied when Ferrari ran my numbers. My watts-per-kilogram for that test was 6.8—higher than I'd ever scored before; higher than Ferrari's magic 6.7 Tour-winning number. I don't mean to imply that it meant I could win the Tour (it was a short test), but it was a good sign. I was in the best shape of my life.

Tests on Monzuno, like the ones on Col de la Madone, were a huge deal in our little world, equivalent to race results, maybe even more important. Some people liked to brag about their test climbs, but I told Haven and no one else. Unfortunately, Ferrari wasn't quite as discreet. When I greeted Lance at the team training camp a few days later, he responded by giving me a funny look.

"Monzuno, huh? Guess you're the big man, now, Tyler."

It got worse the next morning. We'd had our blood drawn and spun to test hematocrit. Mine had come back at 49.7. Normally, that number is kept private, between the rider and the doctor. Not in this case.

"Well, if it isn't Mister Forty-Fucking-Nine-Point-Seven," Lance said. "I think you'll be pulling all day today."

Meaning I would ride at the front of the group, the toughest spot, to exhaust me and push my hematocrit down.

That evening, Johan gave me a short, condescending lecture about being careful. I should not be so close to 50. It became the theme of camp. Lance's wife, Kristin, even made a comment in passing: *I hear you've got some big numbers there, Tyler.*

I was dumbstruck. I knew I'd played by the rules. Yes, my hematocrit was a bit high, but no higher than Lance's often was—and now I was getting scolded by Johan, by Kristin? My Monzuno test wasn't some fluke—it was improvement, hard work, being professional. I'd earned it. And I wasn't being reckless: if a tester had shown up, I would not have tested positive; I wasn't a loose cannon. But I knew deep down that this wasn't really about the hematocrit or the record. It was about Lance feeling threatened.

My breaking Lance's record on the Monzuno—*not normal.*

He would say it with absolute certainty, but he was ignoring the biggest fact of all: that Lance's performance in the Tour was *never* normal. It's not normal to ride away from people and not even realize it, as he did on Sestrière in the 1999 Tour. It's not normal to crush Pantani on Ventoux in the 2000 Tour. Nothing was normal in our world. But in Lance's mind, "normal" meant himself winning.

I once heard Tony Rominger, a top professional who was also one of Ferrari's clients, talk about the difficulties of competing during the EPO era. Rominger said the problem was this: "Now everybody thinks they are a champion."

I think this statement is deeply true, and Lance is Exhibit A. Because of his character, because of his comeback from cancer, Lance believed in his bones that, if he worked hard, he was entitled to win every single race. Now, Lance is one hell of a bike racer, Edgar or no Edgar. But here he was wrong, because sports don't work that way. The reason we love them—the reason I got involved in the first place—is that they're unpredictable, surprising, human. To me, that turned out to be Lance's problem: he couldn't let go of this idea that he was destined to be a champion, and he couldn't let go of the power that allowed him to control his performance so precisely. It's the oldest paradox: Lance could withstand just about anything, but he couldn't withstand the possibility of losing. And that, in my opinion, is not normal.*

Though if Lance is Exhibit A, I might be Exhibit B. I saw my numbers. I saw the look in Ferrari's eyes. I remembered what Pedro had told me years before. And quietly, though like the others I was standing on a foundation that was anything but solid, I started to believe: maybe I was destined to be a champion, too.

Normally, we skipped the Tour of Switzerland, because of its timing. It was usually scheduled two weeks from the start of the Tour de France, which was a problem, because it limited our use of Edgar before the Tour. The 2001

* Armstrong had a new reason to be serious. In the spring of 2001, Tailwind Sports (the management company co-owned by Armstrong that ran Postal) approached SCA Promotions, a company that insures sports and event promotions—for example, million-dollar half-court basketball shots. The idea was to have SCA insure bonuses that Tailwind would pay Armstrong if he won the Tour from 2001 through 2004. Because the odds of Armstrong winning a record six consecutive Tours were considered remote, the arrangement resembled a bet. Tailwind paid SCA $420,000; in exchange, SCA and its partners agreed to fund Armstrong's escalating schedule of bonuses covering the 2001–2004 Tours. The contract called for Armstrong to be paid $3 million if he won two consecutive additional Tours, $6 million if he won three, and $10 million if he won all four, for a total potential payoff of $19 million.

edition, however, contained a unique feature: an uphill time trial that closely resembled a key stage of the upcoming Tour. So Lance and Johan decided we would ride the race; early in the season, Johan had told me that I would be the team leader.

So I prepared in the usual fashion, training hard and using Edgar to make sure my levels were good. A couple days before the race, I stopped using Edgar altogether. Despite Ferrari's assurances, I wasn't in the mood to take chances. I wasn't about to risk carrying EPO during a race, particularly now that the authorities were using the new EPO test.

What I didn't know, however, was that Lance had no intention of racing the Tour of Switzerland at anything less than his top form. It turned out Lance and Ferrari had worked out their own plan; Ferrari advised Lance to sleep in an altitude tent and to microdose Edgar in the vein, 800 units a night. This would keep his hematocrit high and also beat the new EPO test, which worked by comparing ratios of natural and synthetic EPO. The altitude tent would create more natural EPO, helping to balance out any synthetic EPO that might linger. It was a classic Ferrari move—simple, elegant, and not offered to anybody on the team except Lance.

In the prologue, Lance and I were pretty close—he beat me by five seconds. But as the race went on, Lance stayed strong and I faded. By the time we got to the uphill time trial on stage 8, Lance was well positioned in third place; I was in 22nd place, six minutes back, and no longer in a position to lead the team. Lance crushed the time trial. I finished third, 1:25 back. I was disappointed. For Lance, though, it was a great result—his plan with Ferrari had worked out perfectly.

That is, until Lance tested positive.

Yes, Lance Armstrong tested positive for EPO at the Tour of Switzerland. I know because he told me. We were standing near the bus the following morning, the morning of stage 9. Lance had a strange smile on his face. He was kind of chuckling, like someone had told him a good joke.

"You won't fucking believe this," he said. "I got popped for EPO."

It took a second to absorb. My stomach hit the floor. If that was true, Lance was done. The team was done. I was done. He laughed that dry laugh again.

"No worries, dude. We're gonna have a meeting with them. It's all taken care of."

It was weird. Lance wasn't embarrassed; he wasn't horrified or worried. It was like he wanted to show me how little he was bothered by this, how in control he was. Questions leapt to my mind—What the hell had happened? Was there a new EPO test? Who was he going to meet with?—but judging by his expression I didn't feel like I could ask them. After our brief conversation, Lance never mentioned the subject to me again.*

---

* According to a *60 Minutes* investigation aired in May 2011, the Lausanne lab raised a flag about some of the blood test results which led to questions about whether they had been suppressed. After *60 Minutes* aired its report, the UCI issued a statement "categorically rejecting" the story and asserting that it had never altered or hidden a positive test. "There has never, ever been a cover-up," said former UCI president Hein Verbruggen. "Not in the Tour de Suisse. Not in the Tour de France."

Armstrong later made two donations totaling $125,000 to the UCI's anti-doping fund.

Sometime after that, I remember Lance phoning Hein Verbruggen from the team bus. I can't recall what they talked about, but what struck me was the casual tone of the conversation. Lance was talking to the president of UCI, the leader of the sport. But he may as well have been talking to a business partner, a friend.

After the 2001 Tour of Switzerland ended, it became clear that I was no longer in Lance's inner circle. I'd suspected it had been happening since Lance's angry reaction to my Monzuno test. But now it became reality. Lance became even more distant than usual; we rode together less and less. I wasn't asked to do a pre-Tour de France transfusion, as I had been in 2000. Now, Chechu and Roberto would lead Lance up the climbs. And if there was any doubt, Lance and Johan made sure I understood just before the Tour began, when they called me on the carpet for something I'd said in *VeloNews*.

It happened on the morning we were to fly to the Tour in Lance's private jet. I was at home, packing my bags, when I got a call from Johan. His voice was low, worried. He said he and Lance had just read an interview I'd given in a *VeloNews* Tour preview issue. And now we had a problem. A big problem.

"Your quote, Tyler," Johan said. "You have to be careful what you say."

—What?

"You need to apologize to Lance. He's read it, and he's very upset."

I was confused. I hadn't said anything particularly controversial in the article—in fact, here's the quote:

"Rather than just sitting up on Alpe d'Huez and losing a lot of time, which normally I'd do—I'll do my job [setting tempo for Armstrong], and then sit up—it might be important to try not to lose too much time. And then in the Pyrenees, if I follow a break [when] somebody attacks, that takes pressure off our team. Maybe Telekom has to chase, and they have to put four or five riders at the front to bring back the breakaway because I'm in there."

This is standard bike-racing strategy: having two threats makes it better for Lance—as the article pointed out, this was the same strategy that had been used in the 1986 Tour. I said it because I knew that Lance would understand I was a loyal teammate, lieutenant, and friend, and that I would never, ever consider myself his rival as the leader of Postal.

Unfortunately, by the sound of Johan's voice, I had been wrong.

"You have to call Lance immediately," he said. "Apologize. Make this better."

I called Lance and apologized profusely. I said I'd been misquoted, that there was never any chance I'd have any ambitions of my own, that I was giving him 100 percent of my effort, no questions asked. Lance listened, and seemed satisfied, if a little grudgingly so.

In the media, the 2001 race was known for The Look, when Lance stared down Jan Ullrich at the base of Alpe d'Huez, then rode off to win the race and secure his third Tour. But for me, The Look was happening the entire race, directed squarely at me. Watching me. Looking for signs that I was going to betray him.

Which was a joke. I was zero threat to Lance in the

Tour. I was riding paniagua. I had no secret bag of blood stashed away, no Motoman delivering Edgar, no Plan B to keep my hematocrit up, no chance. But Lance thought I might. That's why he'd been so angered by the *VeloNews* quote. It was the old rule again: *Whatever you do, those other fuckers are doing more.* And now I was officially one of the Other Fuckers.

Lance has a thing about friendships. They all follow the same pattern. He gets close to someone, then—*click*—something goes haywire, there's a conflict, and the friendship ends. That's what happened with Kevin and Frankie, Vaughters and Vande Velde and all the others. That it would happen with me isn't surprising—it was inevitable.

I remember once Lance was giving advice to a new Postal rider about riding the Tour, and he said, "Remember, these guys are stone-cold killers."

Stone-cold killers. That's how Lance saw the world. He believed everyone around him was 100 percent ruthless. And his way of thinking worked well. It delivered results. Lance didn't agonize or hesitate over cutting Kevin and Frankie from Postal; he simply did it. He didn't agonize over cutting me out, not for a second. Whatever it took to win.

I wasn't his only problem. On the day the Tour began, David Walsh of the London *Sunday Times* wrote a story linking Armstrong to Ferrari. Walsh had done his homework: he had hotel bills, dates of visits, quotes from anonymous ex-Motorola teammates talking about Lance's role in the team's decision to dope back in 1995. Plus, Ferrari was about to go on trial in Italy for doping charges.

Lance handled it pretty well: first, he minimized Walsh's Ferrari bombshell by doing an interview with an Italian paper where he mentioned he had been working with Ferrari to help him break the hour record for distance covered in sixty minutes on an indoor track, or velodrome. (When I read this with the rest of Postal, we couldn't help but laugh out loud. Lance had never mentioned the hour record to us, or even ridden in a velodrome, as far as I know.) Chris Carmichael assured the world that he alone was Lance's true coach, and other riders issued statements of support—the whole thing was flawless.*

The rest of the Tour went smoothly. The controversy gradually dimmed and Lance dominated Ullrich, who was his only real threat. Lance won at Alpe d'Huez, finishing the climb in 38:01, a full 10 minutes faster than Greg LeMond and Bernard Hinault had ridden it in 1986. Lance won the uphill time trial at Chamrousse in similar fashion. Heras and Rubiera did their jobs admirably, and the rest of the team rode strongly, with one notable

* One exception was three-time Tour de France champion Greg LeMond, who said, "When Lance won the prologue to the 1999 Tour I was close to tears, but when I heard he was working with Michele Ferrari I was devastated. In the light of Lance's relationship with Ferrari, I just don't want to comment on this year's Tour. This is not sour grapes. I'm disappointed in Lance, that's all it is."

LeMond received a call from Lance shortly after; LeMond says that Armstrong was threatening and aggressive, pointing out that LeMond could lose business with Trek, a Postal sponsor with whom LeMond had a line of bikes. A few weeks later, LeMond issued an awkwardly worded retraction. "They put a gun to my head," LeMond later told British journalist Jeremy Whittle. "I was under incredible duress from the Armstrong camp, and my whole business was at stake."

exception: me. Riding paniagua, I went from Tour contender to a complete non-factor. I was 45th in the
prologue. In the first mountain stage, I finished 40
minutes behind Lance; I'd go on to finish 94th, two and a
half hours behind Lance, by far my worst Tour finish
ever. I was supposed to be the Next Big Thing; now I
could barely finish. The story in the press was that I was
"ailing," that I had a stomach virus. I played along; what
else was there to do?

Though anybody with eyes could see that I was in no
position to perform, that didn't matter much to Lance and
Johan. At one point early in the race, I was supposed to
cover the breaks—that is, to stay at the front of the race
and join early breakaways, to make sure Lance had a
teammate up ahead. Getting to the front is no picnic in
the Tour, because everybody's riding like hell and you
have to fight your way past the other 188 riders who
want to be there. It was early in the stage and we're going
like crazy, and Johan is yelling over the radio for me to
get to the front, get to the front, and I'm going all out but
in my exhausted state, I couldn't make progress. Then I
felt a hand grab my jersey by the neck and pull me back,
hard. Lance's voice, yelling in my ear at the top of his lungs.

What the FUCK are you doing, Tyler?

As the other riders watched, Lance shoved me forward.
Cover the fucking break!

After that stage, Johan asked me to apologize to the
entire team for my poor performance. Which I did. I
swallowed whatever pride I had left, and I said I was
sorry for letting the team down, as Lance looked on
approvingly.

That night, I told Haven that I was not re-signing with Postal, no matter what. If they offered me $10 million, I would say no thanks. I told my agent to start looking for offers. The question was, Where to go? There were more than a few team directors who were interested, who saw my potential as a team leader, perhaps even as a Tour winner.

But the more I thought about it, there was only one answer. Only one guy who had been at the top. Who could build a team stronger than Postal. Who knew how to help me become the kind of leader who could take on Lance and win. The Eagle. The original strongman himself.

Bjarne Riis.

Chapter 9

NEW START

I FELT LIKE I WAS on a movie set, a postcard come to life. I was sitting in a lawn chair looking out over the hills of Tuscany. Olive trees, golden light, full-on Michelangelo stuff. It was August 31, 2001, a month after the Tour ended. A few feet away from me sat the tall, bald, still muscular form of my new director, Bjarne Riis of Team CSC–Tiscali. We'd spent the last day together talking about the team, about my 2002 race schedule, about equipment, about training. Now he leaned in.

"What methods did you use at Postal?"

The question caught me by surprise, so I stalled. I'd expected Bjarne to inquire at some point, but I hadn't imagined that he'd be quite so forward about it. I'd thought Bjarne would be the cool, robotic Dane, play it low-key. But, as I was discovering, I was wrong.

Bjarne's secret was that beneath his Danish cool he had a wild and creative Italian brain. It wasn't just the fact that he owned this beautiful villa near Florence or liked to listen to opera. It was more about how Bjarne approached the question of constructing a Tour-winning team. He was open to new ideas, he wanted to hear what I thought about nutrition, training, uniforms, everything. I liked him enough that I'd taken a pay cut to ride for him, in part because, unlike Johan and Lance, Bjarne didn't act as if he had all the answers. If riding for Postal had felt like being in the army—shut your mouth and do your job— then riding for Bjarne looked like it might be like working for Apple—think different.

Our training camp was a good example. Instead of the usual routine (warm-weather spot, day after day of training rides), Bjarne did the opposite. He brought us all to a freezing forest in Sweden, and had a former special forces soldier lead us through a survival course. It was one of those experiences that sound sort of cheesy and corporate, but it really brought us together as a team. There's nothing like starting a fire in the snow to help you get to know one another.

Riis's Renaissance mentality included all elements of the race. Like the rest of the peloton, Bjarne was vastly impressed with Lance's and Postal's strength, and now, as he leaned ever closer to me, he was hungry for the details. Names, numbers, techniques—what methods did we use? At that moment, I got the impression that Bjarne was ready to hear anything. If I had told him that Postal's method was to drink bleach with ostrich eggs, he would have listened. And considered it.

But here's the weird part: When Bjarne asked me what methods we used at Postal, I lied. I played dumb. I told him that as far as I knew, we didn't have any special methods; that we just used EPO. Testosterone. Cortisone. Actovegin. Some guys liked HGH; other than that, nothing special.

Bjarne leaned back in his chair. Took a sip of wine.

"Have you ever tried a transfusion, Tyler?"

I shook my head. Bjarne's blue eyes lit up.

"Oh, you need to do it. You will like it."

—Okay, I said. Sounds good.

I'm not sure why I lied to Bjarne. Perhaps it was because we'd just met. And though I'd left Postal under less than friendly terms, I didn't want to betray them. I look back on this, and the fact that at the time it felt like some kind of moral stand, and I laugh. Honor among thieves, I suppose.

Ironically, it was fortunate I didn't tell the truth, because the intensity of Bjarne's recommendation led me to reconsider my opinion of transfusions. In my single experience, back in the 2000 Tour, I hadn't ridden as well as I'd expected. But in Bjarne's opinion, I had missed something big.

To demonstrate, Bjarne told me how, in his 1996 Tour de France victory, he'd done three transfusions: one just before the Tour started, and one on each of the two rest days. He explained the reasons they worked so well; how, unlike the slow rise in hematocrit created by EPO, transfusions provided an instant boost of around 3 points, which correlated to a 3 percent increase in power. They were like a fountain of youth. Best of all, in this new age of the EPO test, they were undetectable, 100 percent safe—if you did them properly.

He told me all this, then he went silent. He was waiting for me to give a sign. Yes or no?

So here I was, looking out over the hills of Tuscany, at another crossroads. This would have been an ideal chance to say, Thanks but no thanks. I could have begged off, told Bjarne that I wasn't interested in doing any transfusions, and walked away. I could've said no to being team leader; I could've said no to the program.

So why didn't I do that?

I don't have an answer other than the obvious: I was already inside; I knew how the game was played, and so did everybody around me. After the way I had left Postal, I felt I had something to prove.

I said yes.

Bjarne and I immediately started to figure out my race schedule: instead of targeting the Tour de France, I would aim for May's Tour of Italy, a three-week race. Our reasoning was a mix of strategy and practicality: while still prestigious, the Tour of Italy offered a more wide-open field than the Tour de France. Also, our co-sponsor Tiscali was an Italian telecommunications company.

Then Bjarne gave me the phone number of the man who would define my life for the next few years: Dr. Eufemiano Fuentes. Bjarne told me that Fuentes was a well-respected Spanish doctor, very experienced, had worked with top riders for years. His personality was a little different, Bjarne said, but nothing to worry about. Fuentes was very safe. I should not worry. (Here's another pattern I later noticed: whenever anybody emphasized how safe something was, it often turned out to be the opposite.)

I went to see Fuentes at his office in Madrid the following spring. He looked more like a movie star than a doctor. A tall man in his mid-forties, dark eyes, swept-back hair, aviator glasses, linen suits, Italian loafers. Fuentes talked fast. Moved fast. He had a warm bedside manner: friendly, even ebullient. He loved playing the game. He had a half-dozen secret phones; he seemed to have assistants and connections all across Europe. I heard Fuentes would sometimes attend medical conferences while wearing disguises, and help himself to pharmaceutical samples he wanted to try out on athletes. In police recordings, Fuentes called himself El Importante: the Important One. I called him Ufe (OO-fay).

Ufe was from a wealthy family of tobacco farmers, and had an office in a fashionable section of Madrid and a couple of apartments. He was an athlete himself, a hurdler, who did his medical training in gynecology. He moved into sports medicine in the 1980s, when Spain was struggling to catch up with the rest of the world after the Franco years. He studied for a time in East Germany and Poland, then came home to help Spain succeed at the 1992 Barcelona Olympics. By the time I met him, he was in the prime of his career, having already worked with all the big Spanish teams, ONCE, Amaya Seguros, and Kelme. Unlike Ferrari, who had to worry constantly about the Italian police, Ufe had the advantage of living in a system that tolerated doping; racers used to say you could tape EPO syringes to your forehead and you wouldn't get busted in Spain.

There's a story told about Ufe from the 1991 Tour of Spain. He was traveling in a plane to the Canary Islands, the site of the final stages. Some journalists were with him, and they noticed a small cooler on his lap. They inquired, What's in the cooler? "The key to victory," Ufe said. That year, one of his riders, Melcior Mauri, won the race. In five previous grand tours, Mauri had placed no higher than 78th.

Jörg Jaksche, a great rider (a winner of Paris–Nice, 16th in the Tour), met Ufe around the time I started working with him. Jörg's story about meeting Fuentes is probably pretty typical. You didn't meet Fuentes so much as experience him.

JÖRG JAKSCHE: Fuentes asked me to fly down to the Canary Islands. He met me at the airport in the kind of beat-up Land Cruiser that only very rich people drive. He liked having an aura, standing a little ways off in the fog. But when he spoke, he was very clear, very convincing. In the first few minutes he'd explained his expertise; told me he'd trained in East Germany; told me he worked with the top soccer teams; etc. He was like a great salesman. Then, as we're driving, he starts going through the menu of what is possible—testosterone, EPO, transfusions, insulin, HGH, etc. I told him I was interested in doing the minimum, no risk. Then Fuentes reaches into a cardboard box on the seat between us and pulls out some tablets. They were in foil packets, and he pops one out with his thumb and holds it up to me. It looked like a piece of candy. "These are Russian anabolics," he says. "Undetectable. Want one?" I said no thanks. "Fine!" he says, and he throws it up and catches it in his mouth, and swallows it, just like that. I was amazed!

Fuentes is a little crazy, but he is definitely a genius. He knew what to do, and he knew how to avoid getting caught. And he told me several times during our relationship that what we were doing was perfectly legal—and he turned out to be right about that, at least in Spain. Besides, once you're dealing with him, you just have to trust. You're inside his system, and there's no one to check with, to be sure. Fuentes is the father, he is the authority in this world, and so you're in a position where you have to believe. You really don't have much of a choice.

From my first visit to Ufe, I made it clear: I wasn't interested in the bells and whistles. I just wanted him to provide me with testosterone and Edgar, and to handle the transfusions. Ufe agreed—he was always very agreeable. It would be safe, easy, no problem at all. Ufe charged a fee for each transfusion, a fee for *medicación* (EPO and testosterone), plus a schedule of *primas*—bonuses that I would pay him if I won a stage of a grand tour or a big race. The *primas* weren't small: 50,000 euros to win the Tour de France, 30,000 if I made the podium; 30,000 if I won the Tour of Italy, 20,000 for podium; and 30,000 for winning a World Cup race.

Ufe introduced me to his assistant, José Luis Merino Batres, a polite snowy-haired, seventyish gentleman who was chief of hematology at La Princesa, a Madrid hospital. After I had given my first bag of blood, Batres asked me what code name I'd like to use. He suggested I choose the name of my dog. I didn't want to do that—by now, Tugboat was well known in the cycling world—so I chose 4142, the last four digits of the phone number of Jeff Buell, my best friend growing up back in Marblehead. Figuring I needed a code name for Ufe as well, I decided to call him Sam. I decided to call Batres Nick. Sam and Nick: my new assistants.

The planning started right away. The goal was to have two blood bags ready for the Tour of Italy, and perhaps for the Tour de France as well. (And since the term "blood bags" is a bit gross, we'll call them BBs from now on.)

BB logistics are complicated by the fact that blood cells are alive; they can survive outside your body for about twenty-eight days. My first transfusion in 2000 had been the simplest kind: take one BB out, put it in the fridge for four weeks, then put it back in during a race. To get multiple bags ready, however, was a lot more complicated. You couldn't take two or three BBs out four weeks before the race, because the blood loss would cripple your training. The method that had evolved solved this problem through simple rotation: taking out fresh BBs while reinfusing the stored BBs back into your body. This method ensured a fresh supply of BBs in the fridge while also keeping your body topped up and capable of hard training. We swapped them out every twenty-five days or so.

For example, if you wanted three BBs for the Tour de France, you would begin ten weeks before the race, and your plan might look like this:

10 WKS BEFORE	6 WKS BEFORE	2 WKS BEFORE	RACE
1 BB OUT	2 BBs OUT, THEN 1 BB IN	3 BBs OUT, THEN 2 IN	3 BBs IN (1 PER WEEK)

Ufe taught me that each individual transfusion had to be done in careful order: (1) take out the new BBs; (2) reinfuse the stored BBs. This was to avoid filling the new BBs with old red blood cells that had already aged in the refrigerator. Freshness was everything. In fact, that's what we called it—refreshing the BBs. Ufe also taught me about the danger of echo-positives: that's when you test positive because you reinfuse a BB containing a banned substance. So you had to be careful that you weren't glowing when you banked any BBs, because giving a BB is the risk equivalent of taking a drug test. He offered me what he called *polvo*—a gray powder that you could put under your fingernail if you were asked to test while you were glowing. Put the fingernail in the stream of urine, and the test would be negative, guaranteed. I didn't take any. I think I wanted to believe that I'd never allow myself to get into a situation where I needed to use it.

Ufe and I quickly developed a routine. I would fly to Madrid from Barcelona, take a cab to his office, and do the withdrawals and reinfusions, then fly back the same day. I wore sunglasses and a baseball cap, in order to avoid being recognized. I paid cash. Ufe would provide me with the Edgar and the testosterone patches as needed. I turned down most of the other drugs he offered me (and there were plenty), but I did accept a nasal spray called Minirin, which is usually given to kids to help with bedwetting (it causes you to retain water and thus reduces your hematocrit). I once tried insulin, which he told me would help my muscles recover, but quit after it made me feel feverish and strange.

Communicating in code with Ufe sometimes led to confusion. When we texted back and forth to plan transfusion visits, we'd use terms like "have dinner," "give you a present," or "meet for coffee." I liked to keep it fairly generic. One time, however, I made the mistake of texting that I wanted to come to Madrid to "give you that bike." I didn't actually have a bike to give him, of course—I thought it would be obvious to Ufe that I was talking about a BB. But when I arrived in his office, Ufe excitedly told me how much he was looking forward to getting his new bike. I didn't have the heart to tell him that I'd just been talking in code. The next trip, I brought him one of my extra training bikes, a Cervélo Soloist. (I'm glad I never texted that I was going to "give him a car.")

As time went by, I noticed that Ufe was often late, forcing me to spend an hour or more in the café before I got his text message. He gave me his full attention when we were together, but he always seemed jittery and in a rush. As time went on, he turned me over more and more to Nick. I enjoyed dealing with Nick, though his forgetfulness occasionally gave me pause. He kept having to ask me my BB code name. I was 4142, right?

Cuatro-uno, cuatro-dos. Sí.

The constant traveling from Girona to Madrid was stressful. Though Ufe gave me a prescription for carrying Edgar (Haven, menstrual troubles), and though I had a small cooler bag that fit nicely in the bottom of my carry-on, I hated doing it. Security had tightened since 9/11; I was more recognizable now, and each time I stood in a security line I went into a full-body sweat. Doing the BB shuttle, standing in line at airports, getting stuck in traffic, wasting valuable training time, I sometimes found myself missing the well-oiled Postal machine.

Then there was the more practical matter of explaining the trips to my friends. Girona is not a big town, and bike racers get to know each other's schedules well; it's not normal to take day trips to Madrid every three weeks; it's the kind of thing people start to talk about, that would show up on Lance's radar. When pressed, I said I was visiting a Madrid allergist (I did have issues with allergies). More often, I didn't say anything; I just vanished. More lies. More stress.

Making things more complicated, Lance and I were now neighbors. The spring before my split with Postal, back when things were still friendly between us, Lance and I had bought homes in the same Girona building, a rehabbed palace in the city's old section that had been converted into luxury apartments. Lance had purchased the second floor; Haven and I had bought a smaller apartment on the third floor.

Lance and Kristin's place was fantastic. Opulent, sprawling, beautifully decorated, fifteen-foot ceilings, decor straight out of *Architectural Digest*. It had a renovated chapel for Kristin (who is a devout Catholic), and a large storage area in the main courtyard where Lance could keep dozens of bikes, saddles, wheels, and equipment; and where his posse could gather—not just riders, but the increasing flow of people from Trek and Nike, lawyers and bigwigs and mechanics and soigneurs. If

Lance had been famous before, his third Tour win had put him on a new level: global icon. He wasn't like a celebrity so much as a superhero. He was coming and going on the private jet all the time; trips to Tenerife, Switzerland, and Ferrara and who knows where else. Postal had hired some new riders, including a superstrong ex-Mennonite kid named Floyd Landis. Lance and his machine were reloading, and had more power than ever.

All of which made me tilt in the other direction. Haven and I didn't have an assistant or a fleet of soigneurs and massage therapists to help. After each day's training, I carried my bike upstairs and leaned it against the wall. When my bike broke, I did the repairs myself, or took it to the local shop. I liked it that way: simple, focused, no entourage to distract me. Our days were busy and crazy, but also satisfying. I had that old feeling from when I was a kid on Wildcat Mountain trying to walk uphill faster than the chairlift. Haven and I were John Henry against the steam shovel: our muscles against Lance's gleaming modern machinery. He had a lot on his side, no question. But he wasn't the only one with secret weapons.

My secret weapon wasn't a private jet or even Ufe. It was a short, wiry Italian man named Luigi Cecchini. I called him Cecco. Cecco was a trainer who lived in Lucca, near Bjarne. Bjarne had introduced me to him shortly after I'd signed, saying he could help me reach the next level. Cecco's client list was top shelf: Ullrich, Pantani, Bugno, Bartoli, Petacchi, Cipollini, Cancellara, Casagrande. In fact, Cecco had helped revive Bjarne Riis's career back in the early 1990s; he was the reason Riis had bought a house near Lucca.

Cecco had short gray hair and big, perceptive eyes; he looked a little bit like Pablo Picasso. He also had a revolutionary and refreshing attitude about doping, which is to say, he encouraged me to dope as little as possible. He never gave me any Edgar; never handed me so much as an aspirin, because Cecco believed that most riders dope far, far too much. Insulin, testosterone patches, anabolics—bah! To win the Tour, you needed only three qualities.

1. You have to be very, very fit.
2. You have to be very, very skinny.
3. You have to keep your hematocrit up.

Rule number 3 was regrettable in Cecco's eyes, but ultimately unavoidable, a simple fact of life. Cecco made it clear: he never got involved in the dark side. He constantly told me that I did not have to engage in the risky, medically questionable, stress-inducing arms race of chasing after Substance X or Substance Z, or some Russian anabolic jelly beans. He constantly warned me about Fuentes, telling me I didn't need all the stuff he provided. I could simplify my life and focus on what mattered: my training.

If working with Ufe was stressful, working with Cecco was a treat. Whenever I visited, he insisted I stay at his home, a villa crammed with bustling life: family meals around a big kitchen table with his wife, Anna, and grown sons Stefano and Anzano, who lived nearby. Cecco's life was that of a European nobleman. His wife ran a fashionable clothing store in Lucca; Cecco flew a small private plane; Stefano drove sports cars. His money gave him an intellectual freedom that the others lacked; though we worked closely together for years, Cecco never charged me a dime.*

Every visit began with a light breakfast, then we'd go for a ride together and talk (for his age, he was an exceptionally strong rider). Then we'd go into the stone house where he kept his office, and Cecco would weigh me and measure my body fat and we'd begin the real work, a prescribed assortment of intervals and tests, either on the road or on a stationary trainer, depending on the weather.

Cecco swiftly diagnosed my main shortcoming: I lacked top-end speed. Under Postal, my engine had been trained over the years to be a diesel, capable of producing long, steady power. What won big races, however, was not diesels but turbos, riders capable of producing five minutes of high-end power on the steepest climbs, creating a gap, then riding steadily to the line. That's where I was lacking.

Cecco analyzed my wattages and cadences, and prescribed a program of intensive intervals: revving my engine, over and over, into the red zone for short periods of time. I did a lot of what he called 40–20s, which meant

---

* As a student, Cecchini had trained with Ferrari under the father of exercise science, Francesco Conconi. Cecchini and Ferrari then worked together on an Italian team, before each went his own way. Like Ferrari, Cecchini was investigated several times by Italian police, who bugged his phones, raided his house, and, at one point, charged him (the charges were later dropped)—all of which might have contributed to Cecchini's desire to remain an unpaid adviser.

40 seconds full gas, followed by 20 seconds of rest repeated over and over. These may have been the toughest and most productive workouts I've ever done. He recommended that I use an altitude simulator. Soon, I was seeing the results: my top-end wattage was increasing quickly.

We were a good fit. I appreciated Cecco's knowledge, his wisdom, his dry sense of humor. He appreciated my sincerity, and how I did all his workouts to a T, no matter what. I knew other riders who would do 90 percent of a workout, 95 percent. I always did exactly what he asked, if not more. Every day I would download my training file to him with a precise record of my wattage, my cadence, every pedal stroke. Every day he would read and analyze it, and plan out the next day's work. We sent the files back and forth and I saw my numbers rise. And rise.

As May's Tour of Italy approached, Bjarne and I started to refine the plan. Ufe and I decided to use two BBs, one before the race, and one during. Reinfusing the first BB would not be a problem—I'd get it in the safety of Ufe's Madrid office, just before flying to the start of stage 1.

The second BB presented a problem. The Italian antidoping laws were strict; the police had a disturbing tendency to raid hotel rooms and team buses. Ufe made it clear that he had zero interest in risking a trip to Italy. The solution was found by Bjarne, who noticed that stage 5 of the race finished in the town of Limone Piemonte, an hour and a half's drive from the small, independent, and convenient nation of Monaco.

The plan took shape: Haven and I would rent an apartment in Monaco in April. In mid-April, four weeks before the Tour of Italy, Ufe would meet us at the Monaco apartment, take out a BB, and store it in the refrigerator. Then, on May 17, after the Tour of Italy's stage 5, Haven could pick me up at the stage finish and drive me to Monaco. Ufe would again meet us at the apartment, and we could do the reinfusion in safety. The plan wasn't perfect—strategically speaking, it would have been better to reinfuse the BB later in the race, during the second or third week, when it could have the biggest impact on performance. But it was as good as we were going to get.

So in mid-April 2002, as Lance was zipping overhead on his private jet, Haven, Tugboat, and I drove our blue Hyundai wagon from Girona to Monaco. We rented a one-bedroom apartment in a big, anonymous, blue-awninged building called La Grande Bretagne; it was a five-minute walk from the Monte Carlo Casino. A few days later, Ufe drove up from Spain with the transfusion gear. The BB withdrawal went smoothly; I lay on the couch and watched the bag fill. We stored the BB inside a soy-milk container. We unfolded the cardboard from the bottom, slid the bag inside, reglued the cardboard, and tucked it in the back of the fridge. It fit perfectly. If you squeezed the sides of the container, it felt like milk.

We settled in to stay at the apartment for the next four weeks. I had to leave often to train and race, which left Haven and Tugs in Monaco. It was a prime example of what a team player Haven was, because while we'd done all the preparation, there was one element beyond our control: electricity. We were worried about power outages, which would cause the blood to warm up and go bad. So we decided not to take any chances, and Haven and Tugs settled in to babysit our BB.*

The day of the Tour of Italy prologue I was beyond excited. This was the first time I'd been an unquestioned team leader since college; my chance to prove I belonged. Maybe that's why, in the prologue, I rode too aggressively. Five hundred meters into the race I came into a right-hand turn way too fast and smashed into the barricades. I broke my helmet and lost some skin on my elbows and knees, got up, and kept going.

The race was wild. If the Tour de France is the Indy 500 of bike racing, then the Tour of Italy is NASCAR: passionate fans, crashes, lots of drama. Part of it was the fact that the roads of Italy are narrower and steeper than the French roads; part of it was that Italian racers like to take chances, both on the road and off. This particular Tour of Italy was no exception. Two team leaders, Stefano Garzelli and Gilberto Simoni, were sent home when they tested positive.

Now that I was a team leader and taking bigger risks, it was nerve-racking to see other top riders get popped. One day they're in the race, riding a few inches from you, chatting. The next they're gone, plucked out as if by a giant hand. At first, you feel scared and vulnerable—did the testers suddenly get smart? Am I next? Then, the

---

* Hamilton was not the only rider to worry about this, of course. Floyd Landis said that Armstrong kept blood bags inside a small medical refrigerator in the closet of his Girona home, and that, in 2003, Armstrong asked Landis to stay in the apartment while he was away, to make sure that the power didn't go out and that the fridge remained at a constant temperature.

peloton grapevine starts humming with gossip, and pretty soon a reason is established. In the case of Garzelli and Simoni, word was that they'd had echo-positives. Their BBs were contaminated with something they'd taken weeks earlier. Hearing that felt reassuring—bummer for them, but bottom line, they should have known better.

So I thanked my lucky stars, and not for the first time. You won't be surprised to learn that bike racers tend to be a superstitious bunch, me included. Since there's so much we can't control, we do our best to make our own luck. Some riders cross themselves constantly, some whisper prayers on climbs, some tape holy medals to their handlebars. I tend to knock on wood a lot; or if there's no wood around, I use my head. Then there's the superstition about spilling salt. One night midway through the Tour of Italy, my CSC teammate Michael Sandstød decided to risk breaking the rule. He purposely knocked over the salt shaker, then poured out the salt in his hand and tossed it all around, laughing, saying, "It's just salt!" We laughed too, but more nervously. The next day, Michael crashed on a steep downhill, breaking eight ribs, fracturing his shoulder, and puncturing a lung; he nearly died. After that, I started carrying a lucky vial of salt in my jersey pocket, just in case.

Even so, I had my own spell of bad luck: I crashed on stage 5 due to a mechanical glitch and cracked my shoulder. We didn't know it was broken at the time, just that it hurt like hell. I limped off my bike and found Haven and our Hyundai. We might have gone to the hospital, but we had more important things to do—drive to Monaco so I could meet Ufe and reinfuse my BB.

Ufe was waiting in a nearby café; we texted him and he

hustled upstairs. We might have been nervous, but he was stoked. He was talking a mile a minute. He kept saying how great it was that I was near the lead, how now I would be ready to win the race. Everything was *fabuloso*.

Ufe pulled the soy-milk container from the fridge, unpacked it, and taped the bag to the wall. He hooked me up, and I felt the now-familiar chill as my blood flowed into my arm. Haven stayed in the room and tried to make idle chatter, avoiding the sight of the BB. Ufe explained how I should ride with a transfusion.

"When you're suffering, you must remember: you can still go harder," he said. "You have more in your tank than you think. Push through."

I listened closely, and in the following days, I found out that Ufe was 100 percent right. That knowledge changed my career. I hadn't realized it on Ventoux in 2000. The key to riding with a BB is that you have to push past all the warning signs, past all the usual walls. You get to that place beyond your edge, the place where you've fallen a thousand times, and all of a sudden you can hang there. You're not just surviving; you're competing, making moves, dictating the race.

Now that I was tuning in to my numbers, I could feel the difference. With the transfusion on board, I had 3 to 4 percent more power, which meant 12 or 16 more watts; I could sustain a threshold heart rate of 180 beats per minute instead of 175. Five more heartbeats per minute, and it made all the difference.

The thrill of being in contention helped balance out the pain in my shoulder, which was hurting like a bastard. Deep, intense pain, like someone had stuck a screwdriver in my shoulder socket and was trying to pry it off. The adrenaline of the race helped for a while, but eventually that wore off and I was left with the hurt. So I started grinding my teeth. It wasn't intentional, just a reflex at first. But I found when I ground them really hard—when I could feel the satisfying scrape of tooth on tooth—it helped. I know it sounds strange, but grinding my teeth gave me a distraction, a sense of control. As my dental bill eventually showed, I probably overdid the grinding (I'd need eleven teeth recapped). But it worked.

As it turned out, I almost won the Tour of Italy. But on the last mountain stage, with three kilometers to go in the final climb, I ran out of energy—bonked, hit the wall. I ended up finishing second to the Italian known as "the Falcon," Paolo Savoldelli. I made a classic mistake: I felt so good and so strong that I forgot to eat enough. Cecco later informed me that I was probably one 100-calorie energy gel away from winning the race. It was a good lesson, proof of the nature of our sport. You plan for months, you risk jail and scandal, you work harder than you've ever worked in your life, and in the end you lose because you didn't eat a gel.

Even so, second place in a grand tour felt like a massive vindication, proof that I was the team leader Bjarne had hired me to be. I was instantly catapulted into the ranks of bona fide Tour de France contenders.

When I returned to Girona, I saw myself on the cover of ProCycling magazine—"Tyler Stakes His Claim" was the headline, and underneath it was a quote from me: "Racing against Lance isn't a problem."

Right.

Chapter 10

LIFE AT THE TOP

ONE OF THE THINGS I learned in 2002 was that living in the same building as Lance had its complications. The walls were thick as a prison's, but we could still hear each other moving around—dishes, doors, voices. The inner courtyard, where Lance had his bike garage, was like an amplifier. Lance liked to talk loud; when he was in there we could hear every word. When we bumped into each other, we were friendly enough—*hey, what's up, dude, how's it going?* Sometimes he would make little comments to show that he knew what I was doing behind closed doors—*hey, how was Madrid?*—but I ignored him, kept walking.

As soon as I started at CSC, my life in Girona changed. I didn't try to train with my old Postal friends (which under normal, non-Lance circumstances, would have been acceptable); instead I trained alone or sometimes with Levi Leipheimer, a quiet, intense Montanan who rode for the Dutch team Rabobank. I didn't hang out at the coffee shop across the street from where we lived. I didn't linger in the courtyard. Instead of the gossipy scene of the group rides, I was able to focus on my own numbers, my own goals. My system for dealing with Lance was similar to the strategy you'd use if you lived near a pit bull: Move slowly and calmly. Don't make any sudden moves. Even so, my links to Postal were never far away.

One day that spring I answered a knock at my door and was surprised to see Michele Ferrari. This time he had a different way to pinch me. He'd been downstairs, visiting Lance, and had popped up to let me know that I owed him $15,000 from the previous year. I wasn't so sure about his figures—since mid-2001, when I'd been booted from the inner circle, Ferrari hadn't given me any coaching. But I didn't want to make waves. I talked him down to $10,000, wrote him a check, and got him out of my life forever.

When it came to keeping peace in the building, I had one advantage: Haven. Lance had always admired Haven. He respected her business savvy and wanted her opinion on things. In his eyes, she seemed to stand out from the other wives and girlfriends and, as a result, he treated her with respect. This allowed Haven to serve as our building's peacekeeper, keeping conversations moving, preventing any small problems from boiling up into bigger ones. Haven was good at her role because she understood Lance. She was the one who came up with one of the better lines about him that I've ever heard. *Lance is Donald Trump. He might own all of Manhattan, but if there's one tiny corner grocery store out there without his name on it, it drives him crazy.*

In this analogy, Haven and I were the corner grocery

store. Though I still was making less money than I had at Postal, my new success had brought some changes: sponsors, attention, media, and our own charitable foundation. A few years back I'd watched a friend's mother-in-law suffer from multiple sclerosis, and I'd become interested in the cause, getting involved with several MS fundraisers. Now we decided to formalize and expand our effort, and began building what would become the Tyler Hamilton Foundation. It felt good to give back.

If we were a start-up company, Haven was our CEO. She returned the emails, vetted the contracts, even ghost-wrote my columns for *VeloNews*. She made the travel arrangements for trips to Lucca to see Cecco and the shuttles to Madrid; she made the bank withdrawals to get the cash for me to pay Ufe. It was busy and stressful, but on the other hand, we only had a few years to do it before I would retire and we'd get on with our lives.

For the time being, though, Haven and I decided to hold off on having kids. We talked about it a lot; I was in favor, but then, I wouldn't be the one who'd bear most of the burden. Haven wanted to wait until I was retired. She knew how tough it would be, essentially raising a child by herself. So when the old Spanish women in the neighborhood would ask Haven when she was going to have a baby, we smiled politely and said, "Someday." Tugboat became the one piece of normalcy in our world. Tugs was always glad to see us, always ready for some fun, always willing to chase that tennis ball around the cobblestone streets. We took him on training trips, bought him sandwiches, doted on him like he was our baby. In a sense, that's what he was.

The spring of 2002 also brought the arrival of Floyd Landis. Floyd had just signed for Postal, but he didn't seem to fit in with the rest of the guys. While the other Postal riders were in the Hincapie mode, quiet and obedient and neutral, Landis was different. He was from Pennsylvania, an ex-Mennonite with a deeply irreverent sense of humor, a fantastic work ethic, and an unbreakable habit of questioning everything. He didn't see the sense of spending much money on a place to live, so he lived in a small college-style apartment in Girona's new section; he liked to commute to town on his skateboard. He saw everything logically, in terms of black and white, right and wrong. His parents had told him that if he raced bikes, he'd go to hell, and he'd decided to do it anyway. I guess once you risk hell, there's not much left to scare you.

Everybody could see that Floyd was a big star in the making. I think Lance saw a bit of himself in Floyd— the fearlessness, the toughness, the willingness to question convention—because Lance and Floyd started riding together a lot. In a way, Floyd was my replacement. I'd see them out on rides; I'd hear of them doing training camps together. But Floyd wasn't the yes-man I'd been. Because Floyd chafed. Floyd spoke up.

For example, Floyd pointed out something that had bugged me for a long time: Lance got great bikes, while the rest of the team had to make do with retreads. It was true: each year, our race bikes were kept by head mechanic Julien DeVriese up in Belgium; he let us use them for the Tour and big races only, then after the season he took them and they disappeared. We never got

new helmets, though we knew Giro was sending dozens
to the team. We speculated that someone was selling the
equipment on the side, a fairly common practice in
cycling. It was annoying. While Lance was given a pile of
the finest equipment on the planet, we'd be training with
dated, beat-up bikes and dented helmets. I told Floyd how
one of my Postal teammates, Dylan Casey, had used an
inventive strategy: he ran over his old Postal bike with his
car, forcing the team to get him a new one. Floyd loved
that story, because it was something he would have done.

Floyd and I started hanging out occasionally. He and I
would see each other and join up for a ride by ourselves.
Floyd would good-naturedly bitch about the latest stuff
Postal was up to. We never talked about doping. Instead
we talked about how Lance was jetting off to Tenerife or
Switzerland, or how pissed Lance got when Floyd
decided to see how many cappuccinos he could drink in
one sitting (fourteen, it turned out), or how the entire
team was forced to ride with the Champion's Club, a corporate group formed by Thom Weisel and his millionaire
friends who liked to ride with Postal during training
camp every year. We called them Rich-Man Rides. This
kind of corporate showbiz offended Floyd's Mennonite
sense of honesty, in part because he thought it was unfair
to the team to force them to add value to Lance's corporate relationships without getting paid, and in part because
riding with a bunch of amateur millionaire wannabes was
patently ridiculous. "Hey, if I were an NBA fan, I'd love
to watch the Lakers train," he would say. "But I wouldn't
bring a *fucking ball*."

I liked Floyd. He always made me laugh. Plus, I liked

how my new life without Postal was shaping up. I wasn't a cog in Lance's system anymore; I was figuring things out on my own terms. In a weird way, all this made me feel closer to Lance, in the sense that I could relate to his situation. Before, he was the general and I was the soldier. Now we were in the same position, having to plan, motivate a team, navigate relationships with sponsors and owners. I could feel the pleasure and pressure that came from carrying people's hopes.

I also felt the fear. Especially that summer, when I had my first-ever encounter with the trolls—the journalists who pull you into the muck of doping scandals. Up until this point, my image was always that of a clean rider, never linked to any whisper of doping. This ended when Prentice Steffen, our doctor from the early Postal days, told a Dutch journalist his story about the Tour of Switzerland back in 1996, where Steffen claimed that Marty Jemison and I had approached him asking about doping products.

The article appeared in a Dutch newspaper, and it caused our carefully constructed world to tremble. In the space of a single quote from a guy I hadn't seen in years, I was now tarnished. Never mind that I didn't remember the incident the same way, never mind that Marty didn't either—sponsors were worried, the team was worried. All the careful measures we'd taken for secrecy—the sneaking around, the code words, the scraping of labels and the foil packets tucked into refrigerators—suddenly seemed worthless. One tiny story, and our life turned into a house of cards ready to fall. It felt terrifying.

So I did the only thing I thought I could do: I attacked

the messenger. I spoke with reporters and said I was a victim of a groundless, vicious smear. I speculated about Steffen's motives. I pointed out that he'd had his own struggles with recreational drugs (which happened to be true; he'd had some problems and overcome them). I said it was a case of sour grapes.

I was learning: when the accusations come, hit back twice as hard.

In July 2002, I rode the Tour de France, and watched Lance cruise to his fourth and easiest victory. He was helped by the fact that Ullrich was home with a knee injury and a suspension (he'd gotten popped for the recreational drug ecstasy). Pantani and the Italians were tangled up in a series of doping scandals, and the French were still struggling due in part to their nation's strict testing. Even so, Postal's domination was impressive. I saw George Hincapie—big, tall, non-climber George— lead the peloton up the steep climb on the Aubisque. Floyd, the new guy, was ungodly strong. To my eye it looked like the entire team was doing multiple BBs.

When it came to my own BBs, the system was at once simple and complicated. It was simple because few people were involved—just me and Ufe, basically. It was complicated because we had to be sneaky. Before the Tour, Ufe would figure out the times and places for our meet-ups. We usually did the BBs on the Tour's two rest days, always in hotels. Ufe was good at picking middle-of-the-road hotels: never too nice, and never too shabby. He would tell me the names of the hotels before the Tour when I saw him in Madrid, and I would keep the names

on a scrap of paper in my wallet, along with the number
of Ufe's latest secret phone (he was always changing
numbers). The morning we were to meet, Ufe would
send me a text on my secret phone, the prepaid kind I
bought that was only used with him. The messages would
be one sentence like "The drive is 167 kilometers long,"
or "The address of the restaurant is 167 Champs-Élysées."
The words were complete nonsense; all that mattered was
the number. It meant he'd be waiting in room 167 of our
prearranged hotel, with my BB on ice in a picnic cooler.

I never took a team car; usually Haven would drive me
in our car. I wore my usual undercover outfit: street
clothes, sunglasses, baseball cap pulled low. We would
park in the back of the hotel and go in the service
entrance, avoiding lobbies at all costs. (That was one of
the drawbacks of being semi-famous in Europe: if a journalist spotted me, it could be a disaster.) Normally, I hated
walking fast, but I sure did it now: full steam, head down,
up the stairs, through the halls, tap lightly on the door,
heart beating a mile a minute. When Ufe opened the
door, I felt like hugging him.

I'm sure I wasn't the only one making these secret BB
missions, but you never would have known it from reading the papers. As was becoming the pattern, the Tour
was almost entirely free of any doping scandal: zero riders tested positive. The only incident was when Edita
Rumsiene, the wife of the third-place finisher,
Raimondas Rumsas, was found to be carrying a cache of
EPO, corticoids, testosterone, anabolics, and HGH in the
trunk of her car. She gamely claimed they were for her
mother (who must've been quite a racer). Rumsas kept his

podium spot, proving (1) that the UCI was still not serious about punishing anybody and (2) that it was possible to microdose a boatload of drugs during the Tour and not get caught.

My Tour de France went pretty well. Since I had been team leader for the Tour of Italy, my job was to support team leaders Frenchman Laurent Jalabert and Spaniard Carlos Sastre. I used two BBs and rode the race with the A students, finishing a more than respectable 15th. Mostly, I watched and learned.

Watching Lance in the Tour, I couldn't help but wonder about what methods he was now using. I already knew a fair amount—I figured it was a combination of transfusions and microdosing with EPO. But to me that didn't explain everything. It didn't explain the big improvement Lance made each July. It happened every year. One month before the Tour, Lance would be at a fairly normal level for him. Then, in the space of two or three weeks, he would be in a different league, adding another 3 or 4 per cent. In the 2002 Tour, it got to the point that his superiority was almost embarrassing.

He showed it on stage 15, a summit finish at Les Deux Alpes. Right at the end of the stage Joseba Beloki, the great Spanish climber, decided to go for the stage win. Beloki attacks, and gets away. With less than one kilometer to go, Beloki is in the lead, and you can see the price he's paying for his effort. He's dying, his eyes rolling back, shoulders rolling, in pure anguish—like anybody else would be.

Then, zooming up from behind Beloki like a motor-cycle cop comes Lance. Mouth closed. Eyes level behind sunglasses, looking around, checking for others, looking for all the world like he's going to pull Beloki over and give him a ticket. This was 1999 Sestrière all over again—Lance was on a different planet. The whole Tour was like that: Lance won four stages, was never put into difficulty, finished 7:17 ahead of Beloki in the overall. Nobody else was even close.

To me the question was how. Lance had always been secretive about his methods; even back when Kevin and I were in the inner circle, there was always the sense that there was one more circle we weren't seeing.

I knew Lance had a habit of jetting off to Switzerland to train with Ferrari for a couple of weeks just before the Tour. I also had a hunch that whatever methods he and Ferrari had evolved, BBs were firmly at the center. The Tour of Italy had shown me that. I also knew how Lance's mind worked: to do everything possible, because, as always, those other bastards were doing more. If two BBs were good, why not try four? If artificial hemoglobin was available, why not? In the peloton, we used to say that Lance was two years ahead of everyone else.

Whatever Lance was doing, it's certain that during 2002 and 2003, the peloton was catching up. Good information is hard to keep underground. Innovations can't help but spread, especially in bike racing. It's funny—you often hear about cycling's omertà, which is real enough. But when you're inside, it's positively chatty. Riders are constantly talking, whispering, comparing notes. The rewards were too big, the punishments too mild, so the hunt for the next magical product was too tempting. The peloton was Facebook on wheels—and during this period, information was flying. Talk about artificial hemoglobin was all around, and a new type of Edgar called CERA that was coming out of Spain, and something called Aranesp. BBs were becoming more common. A crazy story went around of a low-level Spanish rider who was unable to afford transfusions, and so used dog's blood instead (he won the race, the story went, but got sick afterward and was never the same). Later, I met a rider in Italy who was on a low-level team—the equivalent of Double-A minor leagues in baseball—who was doing blood transfusions. That's how quickly it spread; in a few years, a technique that was once cutting edge was trickling down to the sport's lower levels.

The bigger gossip on everybody's mind was that Jan Ullrich was coming back. After his year lost to the ecstasy bust, Ullrich was attempting to leave his undisciplined ways behind and build a Jan 2.0. He was spending time in Lucca, working with my trainer, Cecco. Like others, I presumed this meant Ullrich was also working with Ufe—which Ufe soon confirmed (for a secret doctor, Ufe was kind of terrible at keeping secrets). I figured this meant Ullrich was going to come back stronger than ever. In addition, a new generation of Spanish and Italian riders were on the rise, young guns like Iban Mayo and Ivan Basso and Alejandro Valverde. The sharp end of the race was going to get a lot more crowded.

When I was thirteen or so, I joined a club called Crazykids of America, made up of kids my age who skied at Wildcat Mountain in New Hampshire. There were no adults, no official meetings, no dues. The purpose of the club was basically to dare each other to do risky, borderline-stupid stuff: climb a cliff, crawl through a long drainage pipe, sled down an icy run on a cafeteria tray at night. The whole point of Crazykids was to get to the edge, see how far you'd go.

Nobody in Crazykids would go further than me. I wasn't the biggest, or the strongest, or the fastest, but I could always push things to their limit. I've always had a love for the edge, a need for adrenaline. Maybe it's the depression, maybe it's my need for stimulation. But when I'm given the chance to go to the brink, I go.

In some ways 2003 was the Crazykid year of my bike racing, the year where I went to the edge. It was, by far, the most successful year of my career. I got everything I ever wanted—every victory, every accolade, every big moment—and it nearly ended up destroying me.

You could see my new attitude in the season's first major event, Paris–Nice in March. In the past, I'd always shown up for Paris–Nice, that weeklong competition known as "the Race to the Sun," with a question in my mind: Was I good or not? Now, with the help of Cecco and Ufe and Riis, I knew. And I delivered. In the prologue, I finished second. In stage 6, I did a strongman move of my own: a 101-kilometer solo breakaway. I was second in the Tour of the Basque Country, and sixth in Critérium International. In each race, I was with the A students.

The spring's biggest, and perhaps toughest, race was Liège–Bastogne–Liège; 257 kilometers across Belgium that's known as the Queen of the Classics. It was one of my favorites; I'd done it every year since 1997. This, however, would be the first time I'd be doing it with the help of a BB. Bjarne and I marked the course into designated sections, and picked teammates to target specific climbs. Instead of racing the entire race, they would be free to give all their efforts to get me to a certain point, then pull off.

I wasn't the only one gunning for a win. Lance had not won a classic since 1996, and had gotten a lot of criticism in the cycling media for focusing solely on the Tour de France. It was a perfect Belgian day—rainy, wet, miserable. Lance looked superstrong the entire race, though the rest of Postal was not. With about 30 kilometers to go, he led a break late in the race, and was well positioned to win—if he'd been able to stay away, or had some teammates there to support him. But as strong as he was, the rest of us were stronger. We reeled him in, with my CSC teammates, especially Nicki Sorensen, doing the yeoman's work. With about 3 kilometers to go, it was down to eight contenders, including Lance and me. It was the same old situation, like we were back on the roads of Nice: Lance and I looking at each other, our wheels one centimeter apart, seeing who was stronger.

For a long moment everyone hesitated. That's when I attacked. I rode like hell, pouring everything I had into the pedals, and they watched me go, thinking that I'd gone too early. We all knew that the LBL finish is a horrendous, slippery, slowly rising road, one of those final stretches that seem to last forever. They figured there was no way I could stay ahead.

But I did. I felt a level of adrenaline that I'd never felt, a kind of panic, as if I were being chased by a pack of wolves. I felt the lactic acid seep up into the tips of my fingers, my lips, my eyelids. The rain blinded me; I kept pushing. As I neared the line, I looked back and saw the most beautiful sight I've ever seen: an empty road.

I crossed the line and became the first American to win Liège–Bastogne–Liège; the media were already humming with stories about my Tour de France chances; if the Tour of Italy had put me in the headlines, LBL put me in the stratosphere. One week later, I won the six-day Tour of Romandie, and became the UCI's leading point-scorer for the year, the world's number one ranked bike racer. And part of me—way down deep—thought, *Uh-oh*.

Did you ever look at the face of a rider who won a big race during the years when I competed? If you looked closely, beneath the smile, you might have seen something darker—worry. The rider was worried because he knew that winning creates other problems, like a 100 percent certainty of being tested. No matter how sure you were that you had obeyed the rules of glowtime, there was always that niggling doubt that you had measured wrong, or missed the vein, or that the testers had come up with some new test nobody had heard about. Standing on the podium brought a terrifying clarity. You realized that your career depended entirely on information you got from some random doctor in Spain, who might or might not know what the hell he was talking about. So while you smiled on the surface, underneath you squirmed.

I had other reasons to be concerned. I knew Lance was going to be pissed. I tried to be nice about it in the press ("Part of this victory is Lance's," I said), but it was no use.

He stalked out without saying a word to me or anybody else. I heard later that he threw his helmet across his team's bus. It was pretty quiet around the apartment when I got back.

After my win in Liège–Bastogne–Liège, a river of new opportunities was flowing into our little *apartamento*: sponsorships, endorsements, media, and the like. That spring Haven and I were contacted by a production company that wanted to make an IMAX documentary about my upcoming Tour de France. The producers had originally approached Lance, of course, but he'd turned them down since he already had a film in the works starring Mark Wahlberg and/or Jake Gyllenhaal, depending on whom you asked. So, as happened often, I was the next-best choice. That's how the market worked, I guess: if you can't get Batman, you hire Robin.

The film was titled *Brain Power*; the idea was to use my experience in the 2003 Tour de France to give insights into the way the human mind works when the body is pushed to its limits. The producers had a $6.8 million budget and plans to use whiz-bang computer graphics to take viewers inside my brain as I rode the Tour.

My actual brain was quite busy with a set of decisions I couldn't exactly tell the filmmakers about. All that spring I was shuttling like mad to Madrid to visit Ufe, to Lucca to visit Cecco, doing my homework for the 2003 Tour de France. We decided to prepare three BBs, one for before the Tour and two for during, in accordance with the Riis 1996 program. I took a break from racing, and worked full-time on my training. I listened to Cecco, who emphasized over and over that all the therapy in the world would not do me any good unless I was first (1) very, very fit, and (2) very, very skinny.

Getting skinny is the part of Tour preparation that is easiest to overlook. It sounds easy: lose weight. Don't eat. But in fact, it's like a war, especially when you're training like a demon and every cell of your body is screaming for nutrients. I spent more time thinking about how to lose weight than I ever spent thinking about doping: the question haunted every meal, every bite I took.

Bjarne recommended his special technique: come home from a training ride, chug a big bottle of fizzy water, and take two or three sleeping pills. By the time you woke up, it would be dinner, or, if you were lucky, breakfast. I tried everything. I drank gallons of Diet Coke. I tried eating lots of raw food—diets of apples and celery. I sucked on butterscotch candies to calm my growling stomach. Every morsel I ate had to be burned off. (Bjarne even reminded me that I needed to account for the extra weight added by a BB in a race.)

I started to get obsessed. When I was eating with friends, I would sometimes take a huge mouthful of food and then fake-sneeze, so I could spit my food into a napkin, excuse myself to go to the bathroom, and flush it. Or, if Tugboat was around, sneak bites to him so my plate would look emptier. It was embarrassing; I felt like a sneaky third-grader or an anorexic teen. By the middle of my career, it's fair to say that I was on the verge of having a food disorder (which isn't uncommon among top racers). But the truth is, losing weight works. If I were given a choice between being three pounds lighter or having three more hematocrit points, I would take the lighter weight every time.

When I was in weight-loss mode, I wasn't much fun to be with. Haven, for one, was sick of it. There we were, a young married couple in our lovely apartment in one of the most beautiful parts of the world, and we hardly did anything as a couple that wasn't related to my training. Vacation? Sorry. Fancy restaurant dinner? Wish I could. Weekend in Paris? Maybe after the season. And no matter how you dress it up, there's not much romance in seltzer water and celery.

Even the simplest pleasures became complicated. Girona was a city built for walking, and Haven loved doing the daily rounds to the bakery, the market, the coffee shop. She would ask me to come, but I was always too slow. I know it sounds crazy—I was probably one of the fittest guys on the planet—but I walked like an old man: slowly, with little steps. Naturally, Haven found this irritating, and we'd sometimes get into fights about it. She'd say, Why can't you walk faster? I'd say, Why can't you walk slower?

Bjarne and I weren't getting along either. He wanted CSC to have two leaders at the Tour de France—Carlos Sastre and me. I, on the other hand, felt that we should put all the team's resources behind one rider—me. We debated it over and over; I pointed to Postal as the model of how to win the Tour; Bjarne insisted we were better off as a team if we had several cards to play. This argument, which played out over the Tour, showed no signs of resolution. I was in the last year of my contract. In the back of my mind, seeds of doubt began to grow about my future with Bjarne and CSC.

While life off the bike had its turbulence, life on the bike was going well. As the Tour approached, my wattage kept going up, and my weight kept going down. In mid-June, I started to get the signs. The first was when my arms got so skinny that my jersey sleeves started to flap in the breeze; I'd feel them vibrating against my triceps. The next sign was when it began to hurt when I sat on our wooden dining-table chairs. I had zero fat on my ass; my bones dug into the wood and they ached; I had to sit on a towel to be comfortable. Another sign: my skin got thin and transparent-looking; Haven said she could start to see the outline of my internal organs. The final sign was when friends would start to tell me how shitty I looked—that I was just skin and bones. To my ears it sounded like a compliment. I knew I was getting close.

Chapter 11

THE ATTACK

THE 2003 TOUR DE FRANCE really began three weeks earlier at the Dauphiné Libéré. Though Lance won the race, he was tested by Iban Mayo and other climbers who did something new: they out-Lanced Lance. Instead of Lance putting pressure on opponents through accelerations, Mayo turned the tables, applying short bursts of speed, over and over. Not enough to make Lance lose the race, but enough so Lance was hurting, and we were paying attention.

Rather than do a BB in Madrid four days before the race, Bjarne, Ufe, and I had come up with a better, if riskier, plan: to infuse the first BB in Paris the day before the Tour started. The thinking was, the closer to the race I took the BB, the longer its effects would last in the race. To prepare, I kept my hematocrit at 45 prior to the race. I took my physical with the rest of the team, then took a cab to the hotel Ufe had selected: a small, rundown place fifteen minutes from race headquarters. Everything went smoothly; soon my hematocrit was at 48 and I was ready. Things went even better the next day, when I beat Lance in a Tour prologue for the first time ever. Everything was lining up: I was pushing good numbers on the bike, the weight was good, Ufe was ready with two more BBs, the team was strong. The next day, as we accelerated toward the finish of stage 1, I began to feel a sense of possibility. Maybe, finally, this would be the year.

Then, a crash.

You usually hear a crash before you see it. It's a metallic, rasping, crunching sound, like a crushed Coke can scraping on concrete magnified a thousand times. Then you hear the squeal of brakes, and this soft thumping sound—the thudding of bodies against asphalt. People yelling and screaming in different languages—"WATCH OUT!" "SHIT!"—but it's too late. It's one of the most awful sounds in the world.

Tour crashes are like any other, except they're bigger and more destructive. This one was particularly spectacular: at the end of the stage, a tight turn, everybody going like hell, fighting for position. One bad move—in this case a French rider cutting off a Spanish rider——triggers the whole chain reaction. From a distance, it looks like a bomb goes off in the peloton. I was smack in the middle of it, unable to stop, to turn, to do anything but tense up and get ready to take it. I hit the pile, stopped dead, and was whipped to the ground. As I hit the pavement, my world exploded in stars; I heard a crack. My shoulder.

Fuck.

I crossed the finish line with my left arm hanging limp, dead. X-rays confirmed a double fracture of the collarbone, a neat V-shaped crack. More out of reflex than anything, I asked if continuing the race was a possibility, and the doctor didn't hesitate. *Ce n'est pas possible*, he said. Impossible.

Headlines flashed around the world: *Hamilton Out*. Riders break collarbones often, and the protocol was clear: one or two weeks off the bike, no question. It was devastating. All that work, all that preparation, all that risk. The IMAX film, the sponsors, the team—all of it gone, over. Bjarne and I both had tears in our eyes.

I asked a second doctor: What did he think?

Impossible.

I asked a third doctor—and got a glint of hope. He said that while the bone was clearly fractured, it was stable. There was a chance. I decided to try.

The next morning, with some deep breaths and some painful contortions, I was able to put my jersey on. CSC's trainer put a couple of swaths of athletic tape across my collarbone to help stabilize it. The mechanic reduced pressure in my tires and added three layers of gel tape to my handlebars to provide some cushion. The team, assuming I would ride a few minutes and then drop out, brought my suitcase to the first feed zone, so I could go straight to the airport.

I climbed on my bike.

Pain comes in different flavors. This was a new taste—harsher, blinding; if it had had color, it would have been electric green. Rolling over a pebble caused a bolt of agony that ran from my fingertips to the top of my skull;

I couldn't decide whether to yell or throw up. But here's the thing: if you can take the first ten minutes, then you can take more. Time stops mattering. In a strange way the chaos and rush of the race was soothing. I pushed harder, using the pain in my muscles to distract me from the pain in my collarbone.

Thank God the stage was flat and relatively easy, in Tour terms. I rode at the back all day, and I managed to finish that day in the bunch. My face was chalky, I could barely talk. I could tell by the looks around me that the other riders didn't expect to see me the next day.

The next morning, I showed up again. Again, felt those electric-green lightning bolts. Again, felt like I was going to throw up, pass out, die. Again, made it through.

In this way, I made it through the first week. It didn't hurt any less, but I felt my body and mind adapting to the task. People started paying attention; it became a small sensation. The IMAX producers were over the moon— *talk about brain power*, they kept saying. I had to remind people to please stop patting me on the back; it hurt too much.

The real test was going to be stage 8, a brutal triple ascent of the Télégraphe and the Galibier, and finishing on the most famous climb of all, twenty-one legendary hairpin turns of Alpe d'Huez. We all knew that Alpe d'Huez would be where Lance and Postal would make their move: they'd use the team to burn everybody off with a hot pace, and pave the way for Lance's usual first-climb-of-the-Tour attack.

Three days before stage 8, I made a chess move. Ufe and I had originally scheduled my second BB for the

Tour's first rest day, two days after Alpe d'Huez. But with my broken collarbone, I was feeling weak. I'd burned a lot of energy the first week. I needed my BB now. I texted Ufe on my secret phone.

We need to have dinner on the 11th, in Lyon.

He texted back immediately—weren't we supposed to meet later? He wasn't sure if he could make that work. I didn't back down. It felt like an unfamiliar role for me—the tough-guy boss. I was basically telling Ufe to shut up and do what I wanted.

This is important. It has to be the 11th.

The night of the 11th, I was in my hotel room in Lyon. It was after 10 p.m. when I heard a knock on my door. Ufe came in carrying a soft-sided cooler. He was disheveled and a little ticked off—he'd had to drive quite a ways to make this work. But he was also excited. Talking a mile a minute, as usual.

"What the fuck, Tyler, you are crazy! Riding with a broken collarbone? You are having a good Tour!"

Even in his agitated state, Ufe was efficient. In a few minutes he had the bag out and I was hooked up. Rubber band, needle, valve, zip-zip. Fifteen minutes later, he headed back into the night and I was ready for Alpe d'Huez.

Not everybody was so lucky. On stage 7, a Kelme rider named Jesús Manzano had collapsed by the side of the road and nearly died. Over the following days the truth came out through the peloton grapevine. Rumor was, something had gone wrong with his BB—perhaps it had been carelessly handled, or allowed to heat up, or gotten infected. A bad BB could kill you, because it was like getting injected with poison. I felt grateful to have professionals working with me.[*]

Of course, there were still the testers to contend with. We called them vampires. During the Tour they tended to arrive first thing in the morning to demand blood and urine. After getting my early BB, I was concerned about getting tested—and sure enough, the next morning, our team was chosen to be tested. Fortunately for me, the protocols worked in my favor: as is customary, the riders were given a brief window of time after being notified to produce themselves to be tested. It's not a lot of time, but it's enough to get an intravenous bag of saline we called a speed bag which lowered the hematocrit by about three points. This is where the soigneurs and team doctors really earn their money: they're constantly on standby, in case they're needed. CSC's crew was as good as Postal's. One speed bag later, I was back in the safe zone. It's a team sport.

---

[*] According to Manzano, team doctors had given him a 50-milliliter injection of oxyglobin, a blood substitute. (Kelme officials denied the allegation, saying Manzano had suffered heatstroke.) Later that season, Manzano again became gravely ill after receiving a blood bag at the Tour of Portugal, and went on to make a confession to the Spanish newspaper *AS*. His confession would spark the Spanish investigation known as Operación Puerto, which resulted in the arrest of Eufemiano Fuentes and, ultimately, the scandal that ended the careers of Jan Ullrich and other top riders.

On Sunday, July 13, 2003, the innovation curve caught up to Lance and Postal on Alpe d'Huez. The weather was blazing hot; the tar on the roads was starting to melt in the heat. On the day's second climb, the Galibier, Postal sent five riders to the front and put the hammer down. In past years, the peloton would have shredded, leaving Lance with only a few rivals. But this year it didn't happen; about thirty of us made it over the top with them. And we were looking good.

There was Ullrich, sharper and leaner than I'd ever seen him. You could almost sense Cecco's influence in his relaxed body language, in the ease with which he answered accelerations.

Mayo and Beloki, who rode for different teams (Mayo for Euskaltel-Euskadi, Beloki for ONCE), were opposites: Beloki had sad eyes and a mournful manner; Mayo was charismatic and handsome. But both loved attacking, and both were fearless: they didn't ride for placings, they rode to win.

Then you had Alexandre Vinokourov, the Krazy Kazakh. Though he had the body of a fire hydrant, Vino was a monster competitor: a tireless attacker, equally good on time trials and climbs, with one of the best poker faces in the peloton. You never could tell when he was going to launch some suicidal attack. Plus, I figured he was going to be well prepared. One time, while waiting outside Ufe's Madrid office, I'd spotted Vino in a nearby café.

At the foot of Alpe d'Huez, five Posties went to the front. Heras and Chechu started sprinting—full gas, as vicious a sprint as they could manage. It was the kind of punch that had won four previous Tours, superhigh wattage for a couple of minutes. For a second, I got dropped. Then I got back on.

That's the moment. If someone wants to see where doping affects a race, I'd point them to those ten seconds at the foot of Alpe d'Huez in 2003. When Lance and company accelerated, I was instantly twenty, thirty feet back. Without the BB, I would have fallen further back and never returned; my day would have been over. But with the BB, I had those extra five heartbeats, those twenty more watts. With the BB, I could claw my way back. On the video, you can see me rising out of the bottom of the picture; I catch on to the lead group. And when Lance looks back, I'm right there.

Lance keeps attacking, spinning the pedals, hitting his numbers. But he can't drop us: it's Mayo and his teammate Haimar Zubeldia, Beloki and Vino. And no Posties—because Lance is alone now; he's burned up his helpers.

A few minutes into the Alpe, Lance gets out of the saddle, standing like he does when he's going his hardest. I can't stand—my collarbone hurts too much—so I grit my teeth, keep sitting, and go as deep as I can. It was like those old training days: just him and me in the mountains above Nice. He's giving his all, and I'm answering.

How's that?

—I'm still here.

How's that?

—Still here.

A little math: the leader on a climb typically spends 15 to 20 more watts than the guy in his slipstream. That's why you want to follow as much as you can, conserving your energy for the key moments, the attacks and replies. The phrase we use is "burning matches," meaning that each rider has a certain number of big efforts he can make. Now, on Alpe d'Huez, Lance was burning one match after another.

We sense it, and start attacking him. First Beloki, then Mayo, then I give it a dig, leaving Lance behind. And it works. For a few seconds, I'm in the clear. On the television broadcast, commentators Phil Liggett and Paul Sherwen are going crazy.

"We've never seen a climb like this before," Liggett shouts. "They believe [Lance is] vulnerable! They actually believe Armstrong can be beaten!"

Lance has the bad face going: deep lines on the forehead, lower lip pushed out, head tipped forward. He drags himself up to me. Then Mayo escapes, charging up the road, his unzipped orange jersey flapping like a superhero's cape. Vinokourov follows; Lance lets them both go. I try to escape again, but Lance follows. Now we've reversed roles; he's the one telling me, *I'm still here, dude*.

By the last switchbacks, we're both out of matches; we ride the last few kilometers of the climb close to each other. Mayo scores the victory; Vino is second; Lance and I finish with five others, with Ullrich only 1:24 behind. Afterward, all the talk in the media is of Lance's weakness. But we riders know that they've got it wrong. The truth is that the playing field, for the first time in my Tour de France career, is level.

In the following days, due to favoring my collarbone, I

compressed a nerve in my lower back. This ignited a pain that was even worse than the collarbone and caused my back to spasm and seize up. The evening of stage 10, the pain became unbearable. Walking was becoming difficult. My breathing was restricted. We tried all the usual methods: massage, ice, heat, Tylenol—nothing worked. It felt like an iron fist wrapped around my spine, squeezing.

CSC's therapist, a lanky, new-agey guy named Ole Kare Foli, decided to try an extreme chiropractic adjustment—basically, to try to straighten me out the same way you'd straighten a bent piece of copper pipe. I told him to do it, quick. So he did. I was screaming and Ole and Haven were crying and Tugboat was barking. But when it was over, I felt better. I lost some time the next couple stages, but stayed within striking distance of the podium.

Going into stage 15, the race was tighter than ever: five riders within 4:37 of each other. Postal, seemingly with only one card to play, tried again to beat us with brute force; again they failed. By the last climb of the day, to Luz Ardiden, we were all together. Mayo was first to attack; Lance responded, and we followed. Lance caught Mayo, then set off on the attack himself.

When Lance is leading, he sometimes likes to make it hard on the pursuers by riding as close as possible to the spectators on the edge of the road; that way, his rival can use less of his slipstream than if he were in the center. Giving a half draft, it's called; and while it's useful, it's also risky. Because when you ride close to spectators, things can happen.

In this case, it was a boy of about ten. He was playing

with a yellow plastic musette—a souvenir feed bag—and as Armstrong passed, his right handlebar caught the handle of the musette; the boy instinctively hung on, neatly flipping Armstrong to the pavement and causing Mayo to crash as well; Ullrich swerved to avoid joining them.

We rode on. In such cases, it's traditional to call a halt to all attacking, to wait for the yellow jersey to rejoin the group—part of the ancient code of bike-racing chivalry. So we kept pedaling at a steady speed, waiting for Lance to rejoin the group.

Ullrich kept pedaling too. I saw him a couple hundred meters up the road, and it didn't seem to me like he was waiting. Ullrich wasn't attacking, exactly, but he sure wasn't slowing down either. I decided to burn a match, to catch him and tell him to take it down a notch. It took me about a minute, and when I pulled alongside, I gestured for him and the rest to wait. Ullrich waited, and Lance rejoined us. Then Lance rode off and won the stage in impressive fashion, putting 40 seconds into Ullrich and 1:10 into me, and giving himself a small margin going into the Tour's final days.

That night, Haven got a text message from Lance. It said, "Tyler showed big class today. Your husband's the fucking man. Thanks so much." I appreciated getting that. But not as much as I appreciated the feeling of doing the right thing. It wasn't about Lance. It was about fairness. Even in our world—especially in our world —following the rules feels good sometimes.

That night I met with Ufe at a nearby hotel and got the third BB. Everything went smoothly, but I had a nagging feeling of regret, wishing that I'd done it earlier; that way I wouldn't have lost time on stages 13 and 14. Now that my collarbone was feeling more stable, I knew that I had to use this BB well. The following day was my final chance to do something in the Tour: stage 16, from Pau to Bayonne, including the Tour's last big climbs.

The day didn't start out well: early in the stage, I got caught behind a break in the field and got dropped. I felt blocked and heavy, as I sometimes did after taking a BB. I had to call some teammates to pace me back; soon I was in front again and feeling better.

When we hit the day's first major climb, I attacked and managed to bridge up to a small breakaway. We put some distance on the peloton, and as we approached the day's big test, the Col Bagargui, I decided to attack again. I put my head down, went into the death zone, and when I looked up, I was alone in the mist, with 96 kilometers to the finish.

A solo breakaway is a strange experience; I imagine it's sort of like rowing across the Atlantic. You start off with a certain what-the-hell freedom; you spend energy recklessly, you've got nothing to lose. Then, as time goes on, your mind starts to play tricks on you. Your mood jerks from one extreme to the next. One moment you feel alone and hopeless; the next you feel invincible.

I went as hard as I've ever gone. I usually pride myself on keeping somewhat of a poker face, but as the photos of that day show, appearances went out the window: squinty, puffy eyes, tongue out, head lolling back; I went sick piggy. My legs, though, were strong. They kept churning.

I inched away. Two-minute lead. Then three minutes. Then four. Then, unbelievably, five minutes. As the gap lengthened I felt myself get stronger: I'd started the day nine minutes down on Lance; now I was riding myself onto the podium of the Tour de France. Behind me, the peloton got worried and started chasing: the teams of the riders whose podium places were at risk. I could almost hear Lance's growl—*not normal!* They went flat out; they pushed hard to catch me, alternating leads between the teams that had the most to lose. But they couldn't catch me. Not today. Everything else in this race had gone sideways—the crash, my collarbone, the pinched nerve. Today was going to be different. The long run-in to Bayonne was a roller coaster of steep, short uphills, and steep, short downhills. I saw it, and I smiled inwardly. It was exactly like training with Cecco in the hills of Tuscany, doing our 40–20s. I used the new top end of my motor. In my earpiece, I could hear Bjarne's calm voice, urging me on.

You are destroying the Tour de France.

Tyler, Tyler, Tyler, you are so strong.

They will not catch you.

You can talk all you want about the BBs and the Edgar; you can call me a cheater and a doper until the cows come home. But the fact remains that in a race where everybody had equal opportunity, I played the game and I played it well. I took a chance and I pushed myself as hard as I could, and when the day was over, I finished first. As I approached the line, I slowed so Bjarne could pull up next to me, and we linked hands in victory. The press called it the longest and most courageous breakaway in

Tour history. A few riders grumbled about my being "extraterrestrial," but I didn't care. A few days later, Lance went on to win the Tour narrowly over Ullrich and Vino; thanks to my breakaway, I placed fourth in the overall, my best-ever finish. I wasn't quite on the podium. But I could definitely see it from where I was standing.

Sadly, a few days later, Bjarne Riis and I parted ways. As much as we liked each other personally, as much success as we'd had, we kept disagreeing on one key point. I felt I needed the entire team's support during the Tour de France, and Bjarne was committed to the idea of dual leaders. I realized our relationship was over on stage 13, when Bjarne, in our team car, raced past me to support Carlos Sastre's bid for a stage win. Leaving CSC wasn't easy. When I told Bjarne my decision, we both cried. He said he'd never met anybody else who worked as hard as I did; I appreciated that, and I appreciated him. But I wasn't a young pup anymore; I was thirty-three, and there was no time to wait.

I signed with Phonak, an up-and-coming Swiss team for the 2004 and 2005 seasons. The team owner, a cheerful, bearlike Swiss magnate named Andy Rihs, was the kind of boss you dream about: positive attitude, big ambitions, pure supportiveness. My deal was $900,000 yearly salary plus bonuses. Those numbers, plus Andy's support, assured me that I was going to be the leader for the Tour, and that 2004 would be the year I pushed all the chips to the center of the table.

In early August I headed back to the States and got a surprise: I was kinda famous—at least for a few weeks.

We knew that my Tour performance had drawn attention, but we hadn't realized how much. The next thing I knew I was chatting with Matt Lauer on the *Today* show, throwing out the first pitch at a Red Sox game, ringing the opening bell at the American Stock Exchange. The traders on the floor were especially happy to meet me (apparently a lot of them watch the Tour). They started calling me Tyler Fucking Hamilton—*Hey, check it out, it's Tyler Fucking Hamilton*—until we decided it was my new middle name.

My hometown threw a parade. Three thousand people gathered in Marblehead's Seaside Park; there were flags and T-shirts and yellow placards that said TYLER IS OUR HERO. A sign was erected at the city limits: *Home of Tyler Hamilton, World-Class Cyclist*. A fleet of bike riders led us in; Haven and I rode in the back of a shiny convertible waving to the people. I stood at a podium and gave a speech and received the key to the city. I looked out and saw the looks on their faces—these happy, admiring, smiling faces.

I couldn't stand it.

Don't get me wrong—I appreciated it more than I can possibly say. I was honored and grateful for all the good wishes; it was so cool to be surrounded by all the friends and family I'd grown up with. But deep down I was ashamed. Being praised made it worse.

The worst thing was, the praise wouldn't stop. Complete strangers were leaving gifts at our doorstep; writing me long, moving letters about how much I inspired them; proposing marriage via email, naming their children after me. To ease the feeling, I tried to redirect the attention. When a fan started asking me about my collarbone, or my stage win, I would change the subject. I'd ask them about their hometown, or their favorite baseball team, or their pet—anything but me. Or when they praised me I would respond with something like "Hey, it's just a bike race." I truly meant it—in the end, we're not solving world hunger, we're just a bunch of skinny, crazy guys trying to get across a finish line first. But my attempts usually had the opposite effect, because people interpreted it as my being humble and considerate. It was like I was trapped: no matter what I did, it created more fame, more attention.

I remember thinking, *This is what Lance lives with every day, only his is a hundred times worse.* We were trapped in the same game, and there was no way out. What was I going to do, retire? Tell the truth? Start riding paniagua? The world wanted more, needed more. And so I would have to give them more—keep winning, keep being the hero they wanted me to be.

That fall Haven and I bought a new house outside of Boulder on Sunshine Canyon Road with views of the Continental Divide and a grand piano in the living room and all the decorator touches right down to the carved wooden moose head on the wall. We felt like we had it all. But down deep, the truth was eating at me.

In the fall of 2003, I fell into the deepest depression of my life. I sank to the bottom of the black ocean. I couldn't get out of bed for days. I had zero interest in riding my bike, in eating, in anything that brought pleasure. By every possible measure, I was at the peak of my career; I had accomplished virtually all the things I'd set out to do and more. I was successful, I was rich, it seemed like every door was open to me. And I was utterly miserable.

What people don't understand about depression is how much it hurts. It's like your brain is convinced that it's dying and produces an acid that eats away at you from the inside, until all that's left is a scary hollowness. Your mind fills with dark thoughts; you become convinced your friends secretly hate you, you're worthless, and there's no hope. I never got so low as to consider ending it all, but I can understand how that happens to some people. Depression simply hurts too much.

We got through it. Haven made excuses for me to friends, and made an appointment with a terrific doctor, who put me on Effexor, 150 milligrams a day, enough to get my brain straightened out. Slowly, inch by inch, I felt myself recovering. After a few weeks, the darkness began to recede; my appetite for life returned. Haven was wonderful; she understood and nursed me through these weeks until I felt strong enough to go out in public, to get on my bike again.

One thing that helped me was our work with the Tyler Hamilton Foundation, which was growing quickly, thanks to the increased attention. One of our main projects was organizing group rides to raise money and awareness; one of the unexpected surprises was how many people with MS came to join our rides. Whatever misgivings I felt about my success melted when I saw a smile on an MS sufferer's face, or when I saw them battling their way up a steep climb. Their struggles, their resilience, helped give my life meaning.

We entered the 2004 season feeling wounded and wiser. We'd made it to the top of the bike-racing world, and when we got there we found mostly desolation and emptiness. I think that was when both Haven and I began talking about retirement. About when we could quit this crazy life and settle down and be normal; have kids, make friends, spend real time together, eat real dinners, take walks. Instead of looking ahead to a long, productive career, we started dreaming about another goal: we'd do two years with Phonak, then cash in our chips and go home.

Chapter 12

ALL OR NOTHING

BY THE TIME I RETURNED to Europe in early 2004, I was ready to go again, and Phonak was too. From owner Andy Rihs down to the mechanics, everyone was on board and targeting the Tour de France. If our year had a theme, it was *All for one, and one for all*.

It started with the people. Our director was a calm, pleasant man named Álvaro Pino, who'd previously headed up the powerful Kelme squad. We signed up a trio of Spanish riders, Óscar Sevilla, Santos González, and José Gutiérrez, to complement the existing roster, which included Santiago Pérez, Swiss riders Alex Zülle, Oscar Camenzind, and Alexandre Moos, and Slovenian tough guy Tadej Valjavec. From CSC, I brought along Nicolas Jalabert, a smart rider and a good friend. The sense of togetherness was increased by the fact that some of the Spanish guys were already working with Ufe, who had been Kelme's team doctor.

At training camp, I set the tone: we would work hard;

but we would also be good to one another. I went out of
my way to show that I wasn't a prima donna. I worked
the hardest; I checked in on everybody, I got to know
each of my teammates and their families. I did my best to
make sure that no one would confuse our team's culture
with Postal's.

We were big on innovation and technology. Working
with the BMC bike company (which, conveniently, was
also owned by Rihs), the team started designing a series of
new bikes for me to ride in the Tour- light, fast designs
based on race cars. We'd have the best skinsuits for the
time trials, the best chefs, the best soigneurs. Our team
bus was a thing of beauty: a rock-star bus far newer and
nicer than Postal's bus, with two bathrooms, leather
couches, stereo, TV, altitude-simulation machines, the
works.

When I saw Ufe in February, he told me some big
news: he'd just bought a freezer. This was not an ordinary
freezer. It was a special medical freezer, and along with
some assorted equipment, it would be the foundation of a
major innovation he was planning. Ufe nicknamed it
"Siberia."

Talking even faster than usual, Ufe explained the idea:
instead of the usual method of refrigerating blood—
which necessitated the trips to and from Madrid every
few weeks—he would start freezing the BBs. Once a BB
was frozen, it would keep indefinitely. This was music to
my ears. I could avoid the hassle and stress of the BB shuttle; I could make deposits at any time that suited me. And
instead of being limited to two or three BBs in the Tour,
I could use more.

There were, Ufe explained, two main factors I should consider. First, Siberia would cost me more. He would have to do a lot of time-consuming work to keep the RBCs alive, slowly mixing them with a glycol solution (basically, antifreeze) that replaced the water and thus kept the cells from bursting when they were frozen. Second, the Siberia BBs would be slightly less potent than the refrigerated BBs: due to the trauma inherent in the freezing process, only 90 percent of the cells would survive—not a huge difference, but worth noting. Ufe explained that I would simply piss out the 10 percent of red blood cells that died. My urine would be rust-colored for a bit, a disconcerting side effect, but essentially harmless.

Then came the best part. (Ufe always knew how to sell.) He told me he would not be offering Siberia to all his clients, but only to a select few: me, Ullrich, Vino, and Ivan Basso. The price tag was $50,000 for the season, plus the usual bonuses for each of my victories.

My choice was simple, because it wasn't really a choice. I could either let my rivals use the new freezer while I fell behind, or I could join the club. In a way, it felt fair to have all four of us together being advised by the same doctor, our blood kept in the same freezer—a level playing field. So I told Ufe absolutely, yes, and I expressed my thanks. I wouldn't find out until later how misplaced my gratitude was.

I've never been so busy as I was that spring as I worked to prepare Phonak and myself for the 2004 Tour. There were a thousand details to consider, a thousand decisions to be made. At times, I felt calm. Other times, however, it felt like life was on the verge of spinning out of control.

I remember one visit to Ufe in particular. I'd come straight from a race; I was exhausted and toting a roller bag. Ufe kept me waiting for an unusually long time at the café. I had reservations on a flight back to Girona and desperately wanted to get home. I drank coffee after coffee. When I finally got the text—*all clear*—I raced in, lay down, and Ufe got to work. When I was hooked up, I flexed my hand into a fist, urging the blood to flow faster.

When the bag was full, I hopped to my feet. I usually held my arm over my head for a few minutes, applying pressure with a cotton ball—but I had no time for protocol. I taped on a cotton ball with a Band-Aid, rolled down my sleeve, said my goodbyes, and headed for the exit. Then I was outside, on the streets of Madrid, racing down the street toward a cab, dragging my roller bag across the cobblestones, hoping I wouldn't be late. I was maybe two blocks from his office when I felt a strange wetness in my hand. I looked down. My hand was dripping with blood. My sleeve was soaked. I lifted my hand, and it looked like I'd dipped it in red paint. I looked like I'd just murdered someone.

Quickly I tucked my bloody hand inside my jacket, put pressure on the hole in my arm. I hailed a cab, trying to disguise my condition from the driver, while I tried to wipe the blood from my arm and hand with a Kleenex. When I got to the airport, I went to a bathroom. I threw the shirt in the trash, covering it with paper towels. I went to a sink and tried to scrub the dried blood from my palm, my wrist, from beneath my fingernails. I scrubbed and scrubbed, not just for me but also because I wanted to hide it from Haven; I didn't want to upset her.

When I got home, Tugboat started smelling my hand and getting agitated; he could tell something was up. Haven asked how my trip went. Fine, I said.

Back in Girona, life at home took a twist when Lance showed up without Kristin and instead with his new girl-friend, Sheryl Crow. We'd heard that he and Kristin had suddenly divorced, but we hadn't expected things to change quite so quickly. Sheryl seemed nice, down-to-earth, and Lance seemed happy, at least as far as we could tell.

Lance and I didn't see each other much, beyond occasionally passing each other in the gateway of our building or in front of the coffee shop across the street. But we were watching each other in different ways. The cycling media was buzzing with the Lance versus Tyler story; you couldn't turn around without seeing a website or a magazine cover anticipating our showdown at the Tour de France. In public, I was my usual deferential self, talking about how I was hoping for a podium spot at the Tour. But in private, with my new teammates, I was aiming higher. I was aiming to win.

We started out poorly. But we slowly got better. I was 12th at Critérium International, 14th at the Tour of the Basque Country, and ninth defending my title at Liège–Bastogne–Liège, before which I took a BB. Each race, I became a little more vocal, more decisive. For example, when we practiced the team time trial and guys weren't riding in tight formation, I had no patience. The old me would have made a joke or tried to be gentle. Now, however, I told them in no uncertain terms: *Dammit, guys, get your shit together.*

It started to come together at the Tour of Romandie in late April, where we had three riders in the top six on the overall, and I won. We gathered at the finish, hugging, laughing, having a blast together. It felt fantastic: a Postal-quality victory, but on our own terms, accomplished with a smile instead of a grimace.

Our big pre-Tour target, however, was the Dauphiné Libéré, the last big tuneup before the Tour. Most of the big names would be racing: Lance, Mayo, Sastre, Leipheimer. To perform well would send a message that Phonak was a force to be reckoned with.

Before the Dauphiné began, a handful of teammates and I flew to Madrid for a transfusion. We kept it simple: we stayed at a hotel near the airport; Ufe and Nick came to meet us and give us each a BB in our respective rooms. It felt strange to be doing this all together, like we were back in the days before the Festina Affair, in the days of team-organized doping. I didn't like my teammates knowing the details of what I was doing, and I certainly didn't want to know what they did; I felt naked, exposed. But I also wanted us to race well, so I didn't protest. Once the BBs were inside us and Ufe was gone, it felt great. We headed to the Dauphiné feeling quietly excited, secure in the knowledge that we were going to do well.

It was usually possible to guess which teams had prepared for a race by seeing who did well in the prologue. By the same token, it was possible to guess which teams had been donating BBs before a race, because their performance suffered (as mine did so dramatically in the Route du Sud after my first transfusion in 2000). We had a phenomenal prologue: five Phonak riders in the top eight, while Postal's riders finished 12th, 25th, 35th, and 60th. In the first few days of the race, I noticed Lance looked worried. Normally he'd talk with me during the stages, do his usual intimidation, send a few pointed messages. Now it was the silent treatment.

The big day was stage 4, the individual time trial up our old friend Mont Ventoux. This was the day when we would all be showing our cards for the Tour. It was a Tour-like atmosphere that morning in the start town of Bédoin. Flags, tents, pennants, hundreds of people buzzing. There were lots of rumors going around about Lance, most of them connected to a new book being released by David Walsh that was going to include new evidence alleging Lance had doped. Things over at the Postal bus were tense. Heads down, nobody talking, everybody walking on eggshells around Lance. Seeing their tight expressions, the wary glances, I felt a huge sense of relief that I wasn't part of that anymore.

Around our bus, everything was calm and under control; everybody was doing his job. I was on a new climbing bike—light as a feather, jet black, with no logos, like it was some kind of secret test plane. I warmed up on the rollers. You can feel when you're going to be good, and I was feeling it: my legs felt springy and responsive. We would start in reverse order of the standings, leaving at two-minute intervals and riding alone up the mountain. First, Lance. Then me. Then Mayo.

The lower slopes of Ventoux last forever: it's a steep climb through a shadowy pine forest. Ahead, I could hear the roar as Lance passed by. I pushed, wanting to draw that roar nearer. I emerged onto the famous moonscape of white rock; it felt like waking up, like being born. I felt good: I went to the limit and held it there, then pushed a little more. The crowd roar was getting closer now; I could see Lance up ahead. He was standing, as he usually did when he was at his limit. I could see by his body language that he was going full bore. And I was catching him. In my earpiece, I heard my time splits. By two-thirds up the climb, I had put forty seconds into Lance. I tried to relax—no sense getting excited yet—and pushed even harder.

Riding Ventoux is a strange experience, especially as you near the peak. Without any perspective—no trees, no buildings—distances can fool you. At times you can feel like you're going fast, other times like you're standing still. Now, it felt like I was flying. I could see Lance up ahead through the heat shimmer. For a moment, it felt like I was going to catch him and pass him. I almost did. When I crossed the line I had ascended Mont Ventoux faster than anyone else in history. I'd put 1:22 on Lance in less than an hour—a big number. More important, five of my Phonak teammates finished in the top thirteen; aside from Lance, the Postal guys were in the middle of the pack.*

---

* Jonathan Vaughters, who attended the race, says, "After the climb, Floyd [Landis] was completely white; he looked like death warmed over. I asked him what was up, and he told me he had donated a bag of blood just before the race." According to Landis, Postal's Tour de France team had undergone a transfusion a few days before the Dauphiné.

I saw Lance for a second at the top. His face was tight. He had a towel around his neck. He didn't say a word to me or anybody; I saw him pedal away toward a team car. He looked scared. He'd ridden Ventoux faster than he'd ever ridden it, and we'd throttled him. The Tour was in three weeks and everything was on the line: the possibility of a record sixth consecutive victory, his status as the all-time greatest Tour winner, not to mention the millions in bonuses he stood to make from Nike, Oakley, Trek, and his other sponsors. I knew he would attack; I just wasn't sure how he'd do it.

That evening, three hours after the Ventoux finish, our Phonak team management received a call from the UCI with a highly unusual request: as soon as the race finished, I was to come to their headquarters in Aigle, Switzerland, for a special meeting. I was confused and a little worried. I'd never heard of any rider being called in to speak with the UCI at their headquarters. It felt like I was being called to the principal's office—*Hein Verbruggen wants to see you*. The question was why.

I was nervous, but I was reasonably confident I wasn't being busted. I knew there were new tests for blood doping. The tests, called the off-score, measured the ratio of total hemoglobin to the number of young red blood cells, called reticulocytes. The higher the off-score, the more likelihood that a transfusion had taken place (since receiving transfusions gives you a disproportionately high number of mature red blood cells). A normal off-score was 90; the UCI rules suspended any rider who exceeded a score of 133. I knew that my score, back in April, had measured 132.9. A near miss, for sure, but I was in the safe zone.

Mostly, I was confident because I was sure I wasn't doing anything my rivals weren't doing. I wasn't transfusing five BBs at once, or taking boatloads of Edgar, or trying perfluorocarbons or some other whiz-bang stuff. I was professional. My hematocrit was below 50. I was playing by the rules.

The town of Aigle, home of the UCI, is located in a scenic valley right out of *The Sound of Music*: cute Alpine cottages, farms, meadows. The UCI headquarters turned out to be the town's single modern feature: a glass-and-steel building located next to a pasture with cows grazing. It was jarring. Until that moment, I'd always thought of the UCI as a major, state-of-the-art organization. In fact, it looked a lot more like a moderately nice office park.

Dr. Mario Zorzoli, the UCI's chief medical officer, met me at the door. Zorzoli was a decent guy: openfaced, smiley, radiating a doctorly concern. He showed me around, and we stopped in Hein Verbruggen's office. Verbruggen seemed pleased to see me; we made small talk. Then Zorzoli and I went to his office. He closed the door.

"Your blood tests were a little off," he said. "Is there anything we should know about? Have you been sick?"

I told him I'd been sick earlier that spring, but now I was fine; that I was sure my scores would soon return to normal. Zorzoli showed me the data from my blood test, and he said it indicated that I may have received a blood transfusion from another person. My heart pounded, but I kept my composure—mostly because I knew I'd only received transfusions of my own blood. So I told Zorzoli that his data must be in error, impossible, and Zorzoli nodded, saying that perhaps there were other medical reasons for the result. He told me not to worry, and to keep racing as normal.

Then Zorzoli changed the subject, asking about the out-of-competition tests run by USADA. He was curious to know how they worked, and started asking questions: How did athletes notify USADA of their travels? How did athletes update changes? Did we use a website, or fax, or texting? He said he wanted to know because the UCI was going to be implementing its own out-of-competition tests soon.

The entire meeting lasted forty minutes, and left me puzzled. For the first and only time in my career—the first in anybody's career, as far as I know—the governing body of my sport asks me to make a special trip to their headquarters as if it's some five-alarm emergency. Then, when I get there, nothing much happens. It felt strange, anticlimactic, as if the UCI had called me in just to be able to say they called me in.

When I got back to Girona, a letter from the UCI was waiting for me, repeating Zorzoli's warning: they would be watching me closely. I noticed the letter was dated June 10, the same day as the Ventoux time trial. It would be a few weeks before I understood why.

As the 2004 Tour approached, my numbers were lining up perfectly. I dropped the last ounces of weight: my

jersey sleeves started flapping happily. I rode easy, careful
not to burn too many matches. The last days around
Girona were thankfully peaceful: Lance was somewhere
in the Pyrenees with Ferrari and a few teammates doing
their usual pre-Tour preparation.

After our success on Ventoux, the biggest physical
challenge was how to dial things down. Doping or not,
you've only got so many days of great form, and I didn't
want to waste them. Since most of the big climbs were
stacked in the third week, I wanted to go in easy: to arrive
at the prologue at 90 percent, then reach 100 percent by
crunch time. Ufe and I worked out a plan: three BBs, one
before the race, one on the first rest day after stage 8, then
one after stage 13, between the Pyrenees and the Alps.
Everything was set.

On the home front, Haven and I were dealing with
a sad development: our beloved Tugboat was sick.
Not a little sick, either. He had lost all his energy, and
suddenly could hardly make it up stairs or go out
for a walk. The vet told us it was internal bleeding.
The best-case scenario was ulcers, but even then we
knew in our hearts it was something more. It felt like
our child was sick; we did all we could to make him
comfortable and started him on a course of medicine.
It was frightening to see the change: he'd been so happy,
so healthy. As I left for the Tour, it was touch and go.
I told Tugs goodbye, and that I'd see him when I got
back.

I went to Madrid for the BB and then to the Tour,
where Lance kept up the silent treatment he'd started
back in the Dauphiné. However, he wasn't being silent

with other riders. I'd heard from several friends in the peloton that Lance was talking a lot about Phonak, complaining that our performance was not normal, saying we were doped to the gills, hopped up on some new Spanish shit. It wasn't true—we were doing the same things he'd done—but of course there was no way to prove that, or do much of anything except give him the silent treatment in return. He and I spent the first few days four inches apart at times, knuckle to knuckle, staring straight ahead, not saying a word. We were both being stubborn. It felt like we were in the fourth grade.

The Tour organizers like to spice the flat stages with challenges; this year they were serving a generous helping of Belgian cobblestones on stage 3. It was a flashback to the Passage du Gois from 1999— narrow, nasty sections that were destined to cause panic and crashes. The key to staying safe, as always, would be to get your team to the front and fight to stay there. Getting to the front early in the Tour is not a small thing. Everyone is fresh and ambitious; everyone is in tip-top shape. It's like two hundred starving dogs racing for a bone; nobody backs down. For the last few years, Postal had treated the front of the race like their own private space. But now that was going to change. Before stage 3, I gathered my Phonak teammates and told them the goal. *Todos juntos adelante*—all together, all to the front.

Approaching the first big cobblestone section, the race started to get chaotic. The road was narrowing, our speed was increasing, and the number of riders at the front was multiplying: us, Postal, Mayo's Euskaltels, Ullrich's

T-Mobile team. About nine kilometers from the cobbles, we decided to go for it: *todos juntos adelante*. Postal tried to reply, and one of their guys, Benjamin Noval, touched handlebars with someone else, and there was a crash. We took inventory: our guys made it through, so did Ullrich's, and so did Lance's. But Mayo didn't. He crashed, and was left behind; lost nearly four minutes by day's end. A lesson for us all.

Lance was furious. But there wasn't anything he could do about it. We were every bit as strong as Postal, which we proved the following day at the team time trial. Postal had a flawless run. And even though we had four blown tires, one broken handlebar, and three teammates left behind, we still finished second, 1:07 behind Postal. It was a message: even when we mess up, we're right next to you.

The next day, early in the race, Floyd Landis and I were riding next to each other. I still liked Floyd, and I think he felt the same about me. We shot the breeze for a minute. Then Floyd looked around.

"You need to know something."

I pulled in closer. Floyd's Mennonite conscience was bothering him.

"Lance called the UCI on you," he said. "He called Hein, after Ventoux. Said you guys and Mayo were on some new shit, told Hein to get you. He knew they'd called you in. He's been talking shit nonstop. And I think it's right that you know."

For a second, I was confused—how did Floyd know the UCI had called me in? I'd told no one about the meeting; only Haven and a couple people in Phonak management knew. But Floyd knew. Because, I realized, Lance had told him.

I don't get mad very often. But when I do it's for real: time slows down and I can feel myself rising out of myself, almost like I'm looking down on this other person through a red mist.

Now it all made sense: the trip to Aigle, the weird meeting with Dr. Zorzoli. It had all been because of Lance. Lance had called the UCI on June 10, the day I'd beaten him on Ventoux, the same date they told me to come in, the same date of the warning letter they'd sent to Girona. Lance called Hein, and Hein called me.*

The bike race seemed to disappear. I felt years of pent-up anger cracking loose inside me. I felt heat, rising up.

Lance called the UCI on you.

Told Hein to get you.

He's been talking shit nonstop.

I rode up next to Lance. Together again, a few inches apart. He could see I was pissed, so he opened his mouth to say something. He didn't get far.

—Shut the fuck up, Lance, you piece of shit, shut the fuck up. I know you. I know what you did. I know you've been ratting me out, talking shit about our team. Worry about yourself, because we're going to fucking kill you.

Lance's eyes got wide.

---

* This was not the only time Armstrong informed anti-doping authorities about his rivals. In 2003, a few days before the Tour, he'd sent an email to the UCI, the World Anti-Doping Agency, and Tour de France organizers expressing concern over the use of artificial hemoglobin by Spanish riders.

"It's not true. I never fucking said a word. Who told you that? I didn't say anything like that. Who said it? Who the fuck said I did?"

—Never mind who said it. You know it's true.

A circle slowly widened around us. He was almost frantic; he insisted he was innocent, and wanted to know who'd told me.

"I didn't say fucking anything. Who said I did? Who? Fucking tell me who."

I didn't say a word.

"Who? Tell me who. Who?"

—Fuck you, Lance.

I felt like I'd been waiting to say those three words for the past six years. I rode off and joined my teammates. At the front.

I think it's my destiny to have good things and bad things happen close to each other. Because later in that stage, I crashed. Actually, pretty much everybody crashed. The Tour organizers laid out a course custom-made for disaster. With one kilometer left, the road narrowed and turned, then narrowed again. We were all going like hell, hitting that bottleneck at 65 kilometers an hour. Then kaboom—as if a land mine had gone off, people flying everywhere, bikes crumpling, scraping, people thudding, flying. Including me. I went straight into the jagged pile, flipped, and smashed down on my back. Hard.

I lay there a second, unable to breathe, convinced I'd broken my back. I felt my limbs tingle; moved gingerly, took inventory. My helmet was cracked; my bike was rideable. I climbed on, numb.

With my teammates' help, I managed to cross the line. I spotted Ullrich and Lance; they'd been caught up in it, but looked unscathed. I felt my back, and I could feel damage. Deep damage. I was missing meat on my lower spine.

That night everything began to tighten up. Like a ratchet, tighter and tighter, until I had trouble breathing. I felt little lightning bolts of pain shooting in strange places. I called Haven. This wasn't a normal crash. This was serious. Kristopher, the team physiotherapist, examined me. He started talking about nerve damage, possible organ damage. I cut him off.

"Be honest with me," I said. "Is my back fucked?"

"Your back is fucked," Kristopher said.

I managed to ride the next couple of days, which thank God weren't big mountain stages, to make it to the rest day in Limoges. Then things got worse. Haven phoned and told me Tugboat was dying, and we decided it would be best to put him to sleep. With a heavy heart, Haven loaded Tugs into the Audi wagon and drove north to Limoges so I could say my goodbyes.

I decided to go ahead with the BB, just in case. Ufe had scheduled the transfusion for 1 p.m. at the Hotel Campanile on the north side of Limoges—a good hotel, nondescript, sort of a Holiday Inn. As it happened, Ufe wasn't there, so the Phonak staffers handled the transfusion; it went smoothly. I went back to my hotel room to wait for Haven and Tugs to show up. But a few minutes after I got there, I started feeling bad. I got a headache, and felt my forehead: I was burning up.

I had to piss, badly. I looked down, expecting to see the usual slight discoloration from the BB. But when I looked down, I was pissing blood. Dark, dark red, almost black. It kept coming and coming, filling the toilet like a horror movie.

I felt myself panicking. I told myself it was going to be okay. Maybe just 15 percent of the bag was bad. I'd still have the other 85 percent. I was still okay, right? I drank some water, lay on the bed, tried to rest.

My fever kept rising. My headache got worse. Then I got up to piss again. I didn't want to look down. Then I did.

Pure red.

Then I knew I was in trouble. The bag was bad. Something had happened, either in Siberia or on the way to Limoges: the bag had been warmed up or been damaged; I'd transfused a bag full of dead blood cells. My body felt toxic. I started shivering, felt nauseous. I remembered seeing Manzano get airlifted out last year when he got sick; he went to a hospital, nearly died. My headache got worse, until it felt like my skull was being cracked and peeled off my brain, piece by piece. I got my phone and set it next to me on the bed, in case I had to call for an ambulance.

Haven came; she could see something was seriously wrong. I told her what had happened, but not all of it—I didn't want to scare her. I lied; I told her I'd pissed some blood, but was feeling better. She got me aspirin, did her best to make me comfortable. I told her not to tell anybody. Not the doctors, not my teammates, not my director. At the time, it felt like a strategic bit of denial—*if I don't tell them, then it didn't happen*. But now I can see that I mostly felt ashamed. My back was fucked. My blood was fucked. My entire Tour—everyone's hard work, our big chance—was turning to shit.

I spent the night lying next to Tugs, shivering with fever, telling him goodbye.

You keep going. That's the horrible, beautiful thing about bike racing. You keep going. The next morning I rode, gritting it through a flat stage. Then came the first test of the Tour, stage 10, a slog through the Appalachian-like Massif Central. I was burning matches all day to be with the front group. When we hit the climb of the day, the Col du Pas de Peyrol, things got serious and I got dropped. The main problem was my back: when I went hard, I couldn't make myself hurt. Sickness I could deal with. Pain I could deal with, but not being able to go hard enough to have pain—that was truly tough.

I lost seven seconds that stage. A tiny amount, but it showed the truth: I couldn't keep up. Afterward, Lance and I found ourselves next to each other. Our blowup a few days earlier had cleared the air. Now there was eye contact, talking.

"Fuck, that was hard," Lance said casually.

—Yeah, I felt like shit, I said, honestly. I was suffering at the end.

Lance turned to me and I got a good look at his face. He looked healthy: pink, bright clear eyes, no trace of suffering; he had a glint in his eye. That's when I knew: his comment was a way of testing me. He wasn't suffering. But he got me to admit I was. It was like he was giving me a needle, a little *fuck you*.

I wasn't the only one struggling. Though he hadn't crashed, Ullrich was having a hard time: gasping on the big climbs, struggling to keep up. He wasn't himself the entire Tour; he had good form, but he was struggling to keep up and went on to finish fourth, the first time he'd finished lower than second. Later, I heard rumors that Ullrich had also had a bad bag of blood. I have no idea if it's true or not, but given his performance it makes sense.

Mayo wasn't doing any better. The crash hadn't injured him, but it looked like he'd lost horsepower. He got so frustrated that at one point he got off his bike and wanted to quit. We all were falling away. Lance was the only one left standing.

My Tour ended on stage 13 to Plateau de Beille. As it happened, it was the same day for which our foundation had combined with Outdoor Life Network and Regal Entertainment Group to hold a fundraiser in which the Tour would be broadcast live at nineteen movie theaters across the U.S. I had hoped it would be a good day for me, but instead viewers saw me sliding back, my face weirdly calm. I'm sure they were looking for some fight, but I didn't have any. I couldn't move my legs; I couldn't feel pain; my back felt like it was in a vise.

I kept going.

My director, Álvaro, saw what was happening. That morning, he'd instructed me to go as far as I could, then we would see. I knew he was talking in code: he wanted me to abandon.

I kept going.

My teammate Nic Jalabert slid in beside me. I'd brought Nic from CSC because I liked his easy manner and his hardworking nature. He was the younger brother of Laurent Jalabert, the French world champion, and, perhaps as a result, cast a skeptical eye toward the craziness at the top of the sport. Once, in a 2003 race in Holland, we'd been in a crash and I'd gashed my hand badly on a chain ring. I leapt to my feet and started chasing, trying to catch up. I was riding like hell, pushing the old wall, and blood was dripping down into my wheels, spattering everywhere, when I felt Nic's hand on my shoulder.

Tyler, it's just a bike race.

At first I didn't understand. Then I looked at myself and I saw that Nic was right. It's just a bike race. Finish 6th, finish 60th, finish 106th, did it really matter? Do your best and let it go. That day, we'd slowed down and ridden together to the finish.

Now, as I struggled to keep up with the peloton on Plateau de Beille, I felt Nic's hand on my shoulder. He didn't say anything but I could feel what he meant: *Tyler, it's just a bike race.*

I relaxed. I let my legs stop moving. I coasted to the side of the road, along a small stone wall, and, for the first and only time in my career, got off my bike while I could still ride.

No job too small or tough.

As it turned out, no job was too tough. This job, though, suddenly seemed too small.

That night, I was supposed to get my second BB from Ufe. To save him the trip, I phoned him. I spoke carefully, in case anyone was listening, and told him that I'd just dropped out, and we didn't need to meet for "dinner." But before I could complete the sentence, he jumped in, his voice agitated, talking a mile a minute.

"It's all gone crazy. Everything's lost, gone. So sorry, man."

—What?

"He got stopped. Police. Had to throw everything away. I'm so sorry, man. So sorry. I can't believe it, it's so crazy . . ."

I hung up quickly, unnerved that Ufe had spoken so openly. Later he explained: the courier had been stopped in a police roadblock, and had panicked, thrown the blood bags into a ditch by the side of the road. I didn't care at the time. I was bummed to lose one, but we had more where that came from. I didn't suspect any foul play—though later, when a friend told me that the same thing had happened to Ullrich, part of me wondered.

I went home to recover. I watched a few minutes of the Tour on television. I could see Postal up front, dominant. All of them together, George, Chechu, Floyd, leading the way up the big climbs, the old blue train. It was a demonstration just like the old days before Festina: one team using its advantages to take the race by the throat. Lance won a bunch of stages in that last week, including several that he didn't have to win, in order to send his message: he was still boss. And when an Italian rider named Filippo Simeoni challenged Lance (Simeoni had testified against Ferrari in court, and spoke openly about doping), Lance made sure Simeoni paid the price. When Simeoni broke away to try to win a stage, Lance, who was in the yellow jersey, single-handedly chased him down and brought him back to the pack, making a "zip the lips" gesture.

In short, everything was back to normal.*

* According to Landis, Postal performed two transfusions to the entire team during the 2004 Tour de France. The first was after the first rest day in a hotel in Limoges. Riders were taken in small groups to a room and told not to speak. For safety, team staffers were stationed at each end of the hallway. To guard against the possibility of hidden cameras, the air conditioner, light switches, smoke detector, and even the toilet were covered with dark plastic and taped off.

According to Landis, the second transfusion occurred between stages 15 and 16, when Postal instructed their bus driver to fake a breakdown on the road to the hotel. While the driver pretended to fuss with the engine, the team lay on the bus's couches and received their transfusions. Tinted glass and curtains prevented any passersby from looking in. Blood bags were taped to the cabinets with athletic tape. Armstrong received his transfusion while lying on the bus floor.

Landis said Postal transported the blood bags inside a dog kennel in a camper driven by a team assistant. "They laid out the bags on the floor of the kennel and covered them with a piece of foam and a blanket; the dog went on top of that," Landis said. "It was simple. Once the blood bags are out of the refrigerator, it takes 7 or 8 hours for them to warm up. That way they didn't have to mess with coolers or refrigeration or anything that would alert police. They could just drive to the team hotel, put the bags in a cardboard box or a suitcase, and carry them in with the rest of the team's gear; nobody would notice." Landis said the dog's name was Poulidor.

Chapter 13

POPPED

HERE'S A MOTTO FOR my generation of cyclists: *Sooner or later, everybody gets popped*.

It works, because it's true:

Roberto Heras: 2005
Jan Ullrich: 2006
Ivan Basso: 2006
Joseba Beloki: 2006
Floyd Landis: 2006
Alexandre Vinokourov: 2007
Iban Mayo: 2007
Alberto Contador: 2010

And so on. It's not that the testers suddenly became Einsteins, though they did get better. I think it has more to do with the odds over the long run. The longer you play hide-and-seek, the more likely it is that you'll slip up, or they'll get lucky. It's inevitable, really, and maybe it was inevitable from the start. Maybe I should have seen it coming. But that's the funny thing about fate: in the end, it always comes as a surprise.

When I returned to Girona from my crash-abbreviated 2004 Tour, I set my sights on the Athens Olympics time-trial race in August. The Games were going to be my chance to rescue my year. I spent a couple of weeks in Girona resting up, letting my back heal, getting my head on straight. Maybe it's the old ski racer in me, but the Olympics have always meant a lot to me (just hearing that theme song still gives me goosebumps).

I dove into the usual drill. I trained super-hard, spending day after day on the time-trial bike. I hit the Edgar, dialed up my values, energized by the knowledge that, though it would be a world-class field, I'd have the advantage of competing against riders who were exhausted from the Tour.

Race day at the Olympics was a furnace: windy, with temperatures approaching 100 degrees. As always in a time trial, riders headed off one by one; I would be among the last to go, along with Ullrich, Ekimov, Bobby Julich, and Australian Michael Rogers. The course would take us through two 24-kilometer laps along the seafront near a town called Vouliagmeni. There were little houses, narrow streets, and sailing boats; if I squinted a little, I could almost pretend I was back home in Marblehead.

I started well, rolling down the ramp and firing on all cylinders. As usual, stuff went wrong: the heat melted the tape holding my radio earpiece, and so I tore the thing out of my ear. For a second the wires dangled near my spokes, and I thought, *Uh-oh, here we go again*. But the

crash gods were on my side for once; the wires fell harm-
lessly to the pavement. I settled in and trained my sights
on the three in front of me: Ekimov, Julich, and Rogers
(Ullrich, starting behind me, was having an off day; he'd
finish seventh). I liked riding without the earpiece and not
knowing the split times; I focused on the sound of the
wind and the hiss of my tire on the hot pavement. I felt I
was going well—hell, I knew I was going well. But I
didn't know if it would be enough.

When I crossed the line I was dimly aware of the big
crowd going crazy. Then I saw Haven. I saw her beaming
smile, which was getting bigger by the second.

Gold.

Our world exploded in happy pandemonium. Our
phones were blowing up with congratulations and offers;
back home in Marblehead I heard people were going
bonkers. I could picture my parents: my dad hugging
everybody in sight; my mom quieter and more dignified
but her eyes shining with pride.

Olympic gold medalist Tyler Hamilton.

That night I didn't want to take the medal off; it felt so
good, looked so beautiful. I set the medal on our bedside
table, woke up in the middle of the night, and picked it up
to make sure it wasn't a dream.

My agent started receiving calls: sponsors, talk shows,
speaking engagements. In Athens, corporations wanted to
pay me just to hang out for a couple of hours in an
Olympic hospitality tent. It felt crazy, getting paid to
stand around and rub elbows for an hour or two. But I
took the check. If I felt guilty about it, I pushed that feeling down by telling myself all the usual things. *It was a*

level playing field. I worked the hardest, and whoever works the hardest wins. After all I'd been through, I deserved this.

I kept touching the medal, running my fingertips over it, feeling the weight in my hand; I couldn't keep my hands off it. I think what I loved most about it was the feeling of permanence. Winning a gold medal was something nobody could ever take away from you.

I was getting my massage when I heard the door-hinge squeak. I opened my eyes to see the solemn face of my team director, Álvaro Pino. I gave him a smile, but he didn't seem to notice.

"Tyler, come see me when you're done here," he said.

It was twenty-nine days after the Olympics, and I was with my Phonak team in a town somewhere in Spain's Almería province. Haven had gone back to the States for a friend's wedding; my team asked me to ride the Tour of Spain. My form was good, and now I had a chance to cap my comeback with my first grand tour victory. The race had gone okay: I'd won a stage but lost some time in the mountains. I figured Álvaro wanted to talk race strategy.

When the massage was done, I got up, dressed, and hustled to Álvaro's room. He bade me sit down, and looked at me with big, concerned eyes.

"The UCI called. They tell me you have a positive A test for transfusion of another person's blood."

I almost laughed. Because it was crazy—as Álvaro knew. He'd been the one to arrange our team transfusion before the Dauphiné. Why would anybody use anybody's blood but their own? The test was wrong. No way.

"I know, Tyler, but—"

—That can't be right. Are they sure it's me?

"They're sure."

—Are they sure the test is positive?

"That is what they tell me. The A sample. They will test the B sample next."

—There's no fucking way.

Álvaro tried to soothe me but I was exploding with questions—where's their proof? What's this fucking test? Who do I call? Where is this lab? We told the press I had stomach troubles and I dropped out of the race. We found team owner Andy Rihs, who was at the race. He looked in my eyes and asked if I'd done it. I didn't blink. I looked in his eyes and told him I was innocent.

I went to my hotel room, took a deep breath, and dialed Haven. I tried to make it sound like a glitch, a harmless fluke that would soon be fixed, but I could hear the tremble in her voice, and I'm sure she could hear it in mine. Haven was no fool. She knew precisely how serious this was, and she knew we were now in a race: we had to get this taken care of before the media found out. Once it hit the Internet, the story would be everywhere, and I'd be stained. I told Haven everything was going to be okay, and I tried to sound convincing. I hung up the phone and sat in silence.

This was the moment, the fork in the road. Everyone who gets popped experiences it: that eerie calm before the storm, those few hours when they can decide to tell the truth or not. I'd like to tell you that I thought about confessing, but the truth is I never considered it, not for one second. Confession felt impossible, unthinkable, an act of insanity. Not just because I'd spent years playing the game, telling myself that I wasn't a cheater, that everybody did it. Not just because it would mean the shame of being exposed, or the loss of my team and contract and good name, or having to tell my parents. Not just because confession would implicate my friends, possibly end the careers of my teammates and staffers—after all, it wasn't like I'd done all this solo. But mostly because the charge didn't make any sense to me. The UCI was claiming I had someone else's blood in my body—and I was 100 percent sure that I didn't. Should I ruin my life and others' lives by pleading guilty to something I hadn't done? To me, the answer was clear: *No.**

Andy, Álvaro, and I huddled, and tried to figure out a strategy. We all knew the protocol: the testers take two samples, an A sample and a B sample. My A sample had tested positive; the B sample hadn't yet been tested. If the tests matched—and they almost always did—then I was officially, publicly positive, automatically suspended, and would have to fight the test with USADA, the antidoping organization that has jurisdiction over every American professional cyclist. Our thoughts immediately went toward disproving the test for blood transfusion, which, we were discovering, was a brand-new test. In fact, I was the first person to test positive. Rihs was

---

* If Hamilton had immediately confessed, it would have been a first. Cycling history contains zero examples of high-level racers who, having tested positive for doping, offered an immediate and complete confession. Even those who eventually come clean, like former world champion David Millar, spend months denying or claiming they'd only doped once or twice. Part of the reason is legal, but the larger part seems psychological: they don't feel like they've done anything wrong, so there's nothing to confess.

supportive, said he'd help me get the best lawyers, the best doctors, even spend his own money to fund an independent scientific investigation of the test.

Then it got worse. Two days after the Tour of Spain positive, the International Olympic Committee (IOC) informed me that my A test from the Olympics had also tested positive. My heart sank. This wasn't some random glitch of the test; it was a pattern. Now they had two results, two glowing test tubes, two uphill battles for me to fight.

Life became a nightmare. I flew to Lausanne, Switzerland, to watch the lab conduct the test of the B sample. When the media swarm started humming with news of my positive test, I held a press conference in Switzerland alongside Rihs, and we said all the right things—we'd do whatever it took to clear my name. I tried not to lie too much. I know that sounds crazy— I mean, there I was, having doped consistently for eight years, professing my innocence—but I instinctively tried to keep things as close to the truth as I could. I felt like I was an actor trapped in a terrible play, with no choice but to move ahead.

"I've always been an honest person since I grew up," I said. "My family taught me to be an honest person since I was a kid. I've always believed in fair play . . . I've been accused of taking blood from another person, which if anybody knows me, knows that that is completely impossible . . . I can guarantee you the gold medal will be staying in my living room until I don't have a cent left."

Underneath my brave front, though, I felt powerless. I knew all too well how these things could be handled, if you had the connections. Back in 1999, when Lance tested positive for cortisone, it was handled quietly with Tour officials, and solved with a prescription. Back in 2001, when Lance had the suspicious EPO test at the Tour of Switzerland, the same thing had happened: he'd had meetings with people at the lab and it all went away. Lance worked the system—hell, Lance *was* the system. But who could I call? Who would help me?

No one.

After the press conference, I checked my messages and texts. I was hoping to hear some messages from my Postal or Phonak friends, the guys who understood what I was going through. I wanted to hear some "hang in theres" or "thinking about yous." But I didn't. My phone was filled with messages and texts from journalists. That was it. Haven would be in the States for another week. I was alone.

Not knowing what else to do, I traveled back to Girona. I felt like a fugitive. I wore my sunglasses and pulled my ball cap low, imagining the accusing stares: *There he goes. Cheater. Doper.* I walked down the narrow street and unlocked the gate to our shared courtyard. I was never more grateful that Lance wasn't around. I walked upstairs to our apartment and locked the door behind me. I sat down on one of the stools next to the kitchen counter, and I stared at the floor.

I don't know how long I sat there. A day? Two days? I didn't eat. I didn't sleep. I didn't cry. I felt dead inside, a zombie. I stared at the floor for hours, trying to accept that this was happening. Trying to get ready for what lay ahead. I stared at the floor and tried to harden my mind.

I'm not gonna let this beat me. I'm not going to become an angry or bitter guy. Nothing is going to change. *Nothing is going to change.*

I'm going to get through this. It might take a while, but I'll get through.

I'm still Tyler. I'm still Tyler. I'm still Tyler.

Getting popped makes you go a little crazy. You've spent your career inside this elite brotherhood, this family, playing the game alongside everybody else when suddenly—*whoosh*, you're flushed into a world of shit, labeled "doper" in headlines, deprived of your income, and—here's the worst part—everybody in the brotherhood pretends that you never existed. You realize you've been sacrificed to keep the circus going; you're the reason they can pretend they're clean. You're alone, and the only way back is to spend years and hundreds of thousands of dollars on lawyers so that you can, if you're lucky, grovel your way back to rejoining that same messed-up world that chucked you out in the first place.

When Marco Pantani got popped in 1999 and 2001, he got depressed, and ended up overdosing on cocaine in 2004. Jörg Jaksche suffered from depression after his bust; so did Floyd Landis. Jan Ullrich was treated in a clinic for "burnout syndrome." Iban Mayo maybe had the best reaction: when he was busted he quit bike racing, and I heard he became a long-distance truck driver. In the days after my positive test, I fantasized about doing something like that, maybe getting a job as a carpenter.

But I couldn't quit, not now. Neither could Haven. So we set out to clear our name. It was our old reflex of getting ready for a big race—except now we had to deal with mountains of legal and scientific paper, trying to destroy this test before it destroyed me.

We poured all our energy into the project. We hired the best sports-doping lawyer we could find, Howard Jacobs, and set up an office in our Colorado house. We dug into the history and reliability of the test, especially when it came to false positives. We found that false positives can be caused by a number of conditions, including chimerism, a rare fetal condition that can result in a person having two distinct blood types, also called "vanishing twin." While we never claimed that I was a chimerical twin, the press had a field day making jokes about my "vanishing-twin defense" as if that were the centerpiece of our strategy. The press didn't understand that our job was to throw the kitchen sink at the test, to cast its credibility into doubt. (Law, I was discovering, works like bike racing: try everything, just in case it works.)

Early on, we received some good news: I'd be keeping the Olympic gold medal. For an unexplained reason, the Athens lab had frozen the B sample, rendering it untestable and therefore failing to confirm the positive A test. This was good news, not just for the gold, but because it showed that the lab was sloppy.

We also learned a disconcerting story about a Swiss man named Christian Vinzens. According to reports in Swiss newspapers, Vinzens had attempted to extort Phonak officials before the positive results went public by claiming to know which Phonak riders, including me, were going to test positive; he was demanding payment from team officials in exchange for making the problem go away. While we were never able to prove any causal link between Vinzens and the test, it added to our sense that there was more to this story for us to uncover.

Meanwhile, our friends and families supported us 100 percent. People were incredibly kind: they wrote letters, sent emails, even donated money. A high school friend started believetyler.org; red wristbands were sold that said BELIEVE.*

I was living with so many levels of delusion. On the surface, I was grateful for the support. Beneath that, I was uncomfortable with it, especially the "Believe Tyler" tagline that made me appear like such a saint. Beneath *that*, I knew in my heart that I was guilty as sin—maybe not guilty of this specific charge, but guilty of living a lie. Yet I wasn't in a position to try to enlighten my team of supporters. ("*Uh, listen, guys, thanks for everything but the truth is, I'm not entirely innocent . . .*") Besides, I didn't exactly have to take acting lessons in order to feel persecuted. I felt like I was being victimized— by the sport, by the UCI, by the testers, by some of the peloton, by certain members of the press, and most of all by a world that was swift to lump me into the category of "cheater," "doper," and "liar" without looking at the details. So when my friends saw me as an innocent who was being unfairly railroaded, it fit well enough. When the people in my foundation wanted to organize events, I

---

* About $25,000 in all, which according to Hamilton was never used in his defense. "I didn't feel comfortable using it, so we finally put it in the Tyler Hamilton Foundation." Bereft of support, the foundation closed in 2008 with a negative balance on the books.

said yes. When my parents, with tears in their eyes, told me that they believed in me and were going to do everything in their power to help, I thanked them with all my heart, and I meant it.

Meanwhile, Haven and I were living in a catacomb of legal boxes. We barely slept, working seven days a week, twelve hours a day, racing through an endless jungle of problems and legal strategies. We hired experts from MIT, Harvard Medical School, Puget Sound Blood Center, Georgetown University Hospital, and the Fred Hutchinson Cancer Research Center. We found out the details behind the test's development, including a tall stack of emails questioning why it produced false positives. I traveled to Athens, and got more seemingly useful material—emails from lab techs questioning the test's accuracy. We petitioned the UCI to release the paperwork on blood tests I'd taken in July, during the Tour, and when they failed to release them, Howard Jacobs and I traveled to the lab in Lausanne and dug in like a couple of gumshoes, unearthing the paperwork we needed.

I got better at making my case with the public. I learned that if you're vague enough, you don't have to lie. I said things like "I've always been a hard worker," and "I've been at the top consistently for ten years," and "I've tested clean dozens of times," and so on. I learned that if you repeat something often enough, you begin to believe it. I even took a lie-detector test to help prove my innocence, and passed. (Though, just before taking it, we Googled a few tips for beating the test. Clenching your buttocks, I remember, was one.)

To pay our legal bills, which would eventually add up

to about $1 million, we sold our house in Marblehead and our little house in Nederland, the one I'd bought back when I was a neo-pro. Selling that little house hurt, but we did it because we were convinced we were going to win and be vindicated. Meanwhile, I kept training, fueled by a new anger, taking crazy-long rides in the mountains around Boulder. I was going to show those sons of bitches. I was going to come back all the way. As our arbitration date approached, I felt myself getting more and more excited, picturing myself back in the Tour. This test was bullshit—I knew it and they knew it. I knew we were going to win. We had to win.

Then we lost.

We lost not once, but twice. First at a USADA hearing in April 2005, and then, on appeal, in the Court of Arbitration for Sport (CAS) in February 2006. Their side argued the test was solid; that the emails and other materials we'd uncovered were "evidence of normal scientific debate." We were devastated. I had no choice but to express my disappointment, serve out the rest of my two-year suspension, and rejoin the peloton in the fall of 2006.*

---

* The big question: Presuming the blood test was accurate, how did someone else's blood get inside Hamilton's body? Some theories suggested that Hamilton's blood had been mixed up with that of Phonak teammate Santiago Pérez, who was busted just after winning the 2004 Tour of Spain for the same offense. (This didn't turn out to be possible, due to differences in blood type.)

Dr. Michael Ashenden, the Australian scientist who helped develop the test and who testified in Hamilton's USADA hearing, suggests that there could have been a mix-up somewhere in Fuentes's transfusion procedure. Freezing blood is a multi-step procedure that includes several transfers and mixings with progressively stronger concentrations of glycol with a mixing machine called an ACP-215. Because the cells are alive, you have to babysit

Losing has a way of clearing your vision. We saw how naïve we'd been, how we'd thrown everything into a hopeless cause. I saw how the system really worked. This wasn't like a jury trial—we weren't innocent until proven guilty. The threshold phrase that USADA used was "comfortable satisfaction." They looked at the evidence, and they decided. Despite all our work, it felt like we'd never really had a shot.

Looking back, I can see that this was the moment when things with Haven started to fall apart. Over the past couple of years, our relationship had become more of a business partnership; it often felt as if we were a couple of overworked lawyers who happened to sleep in the same bed. Until the verdicts, we had told ourselves it was all going to be worth it, that we were going to be proven innocent, we were going to wipe this stain away and then come back even stronger.

this machine for hours at a time, and keep everything straight. In a situation where Fuentes and his assistant, José Maria Batres (aka Nick), were handling the blood of dozens of riders, it would be possible to envision a scenario where Hamilton's and another racer's blood were accidentally mislabeled and/or mixed. In addition, according to Spanish newspaper reports in 2010, Batres was suffering from dementia.

While Hamilton has never reduced his criticism of the test, which he regarded as "clearly not ready for prime time," he gradually grew to accept the possibility that his positive might have resulted from a simple accident. "At times, Nick [Batres] did seem a little mixed up," he says. "I always had to remind him of my code name."

It's also interesting that Dr. Ashenden, in the wake of the confessions of Hamilton, Landis, and others, had gradually come to understand doping from the bike racer's point of view. "Before, I saw them as weak people, bad people," he said. "Now I see that they're put in an impossible situation. If I had been put in their situation, I would do what they did."

Now, in the quiet weeks after the decision, we realized how incredibly tired we were—tired of battling the system, tired of losing, tired of playing these roles of the never-say-die cyclist and plucky, supportive wife. We'd worked so hard, we'd given our absolute all, and it had all been for nothing. We tried to pick ourselves up, to tell ourselves that this was just another bump in the road, that we could tough this out just like we'd toughed everything else out. But in reality, we were finding out that toughness, and our relationship, had their limits

By the time my final CAS appeal was denied, Lance was retired. He'd won his record seventh Tour in 2005, and had addressed his doubters from the podium. He'd said, "I feel sorry for you. I'm sorry you can't dream big and I'm sorry you don't believe in miracles." With that, he'd ridden off into the sunset.*

* Not quite, of course, because Armstrong was also fighting his own handful of legal battles, among them:

(1) a lawsuit against Mike Anderson, a former personal assistant who said he had been fired because he had accidentally discovered doping products in Armstrong's Girona apartment. Armstrong filed suit against Anderson; the case was later settled out of court.

(2) libel suits against, among others, La Martinière, the French publishers of David Walsh's and Pierre Ballester's *L.A. Confidentiel*, and the London *Sunday Times*. Armstrong eventually dropped the suit against Martinière, and won an apology from the *Sunday Times*.

(3) a lawsuit against SCA Promotions, the insurance company contracted to cover Armstrong's bonuses for winning the Tour de France. In 2004, after SCA executives grew suspicious about Armstrong's possible doping, the company withheld Armstrong's $5 million bonus. Armstrong filed suit, and an arbitration hearing was held in the fall of 2005, in which Armstrong, Greg LeMond, Frankie and Betsy Andreu, and others were deposed under oath. As

Then, with timing that can only be described as poetic, the sport had its next great scandal. This one, though, involved someone I knew rather well. Ufe.

In late May 2006 Spanish police raided Ufe's Madrid office—that office I knew so well—along with a couple of nearby apartments. They emerged with a trove of evidence that astonished the world. Two hundred and twenty BBs. Twenty bags of plasma. Two refrigerators. One freezer (which I presumed was good old Siberia). Large plastic totes filled with no fewer than 105 different medications, including Prozac, Actovegin, insulin, and EPO; billing information; invoices; rate sheets; calendars; lists of hotels for the Tour of Italy and Tour de France; and the bonuses he was due when a client won a stage or a race.

Now, I had known Ufe was a busy guy. I'd always known he worked with other riders—he'd told me about Ullrich and Basso himself. But the truth was now clear: Ufe hadn't been a boutique service for elite riders; he had been a one-man Wal-Mart, servicing what seemed to be half the peloton. Officially, the police linked forty-one riders to him; unofficially they said there might be more,

the law focused solely on the terms of the original contract—that is, if Armstrong won, SCA had to pay regardless of any questions over what methods he might have used to win—SCA eventually settled, paying the $5 million plus $2.5 million in interest and lawyers' fees.

Armstrong was not just playing defense, however. In the fall of 2006, according to *The Wall Street Journal*, Armstrong and his agent, Bill Stapleton, began talking to potential investors about purchasing the Tour de France from its owner, the Amaury Sport Organisation, for $1.5 billion. Due to a variety of factors, including the global economic slowdown, the deal was never completed. Armstrong remained tempted by the notion of buying the Tour, describing it in 2011 as "a great idea," but difficult to execute.

including tennis players and soccer teams. Prosecutors calculated that in the first quarter of 2006, Ufe made
470,000 euros ($564,000).

> JONATHAN VAUGHTERS: The thing to realize about
> Fuentes and all these guys is that they're doping
> doctors for a reason. They're the ones who didn't
> make it on the conventional path, so they're not the
> most organized people. So when they leave a bag of
> blood out in the sun because they're having another
> glass of wine at the café, it's predictable. The deadly
> mistake that Tyler, Floyd, Roberto [Heras], and the
> rest of them made when they left Postal was to
> assume that they'd find other doctors who were as
> professional. But when they got out there, they
> found—whoops!—there weren't any others.

As worried as I was about being sucked into the unfolding
controversy, a small part of me had to salute him for his
tactical brilliance. Ufe, you cunning bastard! You figured it
out, you used the shadows of our world to play the angles
like a master. Even being conservative, Ufe was making
millions. You weren't just a talented doctor. You were also a
talented con man. What's more, you knew all along that you
were safe, because Spain lacked laws against sports doping.*

* Fuentes's confidence appears to have been well placed. Because there was
no law against doping in Spain, the Operación Puerto prosecution languished
in Spanish courts. Fuentes was ultimately charged with a crime against public health; his defense filings pointed out that all the transfusions he
supervised were performed in hygienic conditions under the supervision of
safe, qualified personnel.

Operación Puerto, like Festina eight years earlier, hit the sport like an atomic bomb, smack on the eve of the 2006 Tour de France. Some implicated riders like Ivan Basso and Frank Schleck (who admitted to paying Fuentes 7,000 euros) would lamely claim that they hadn't doped. Others, like Ullrich, had the good sense to retire (good idea, since DNA tests showed Ullrich had nine BBs in Ufe's possession). The Tour went on, but it didn't get any better: the eventual winner, Floyd Landis, whom I'd helped bring to Phonak, was popped for testosterone a couple days after the Tour ended.

I felt for all the guys who got busted that year, but I felt most for Floyd because of how it happened. He'd won the Tour in dramatic come-from-behind fashion, accomplishing what veteran observers called the greatest single ride in Tour history, a solo breakaway on stage 17 where he outrode a chasing peloton over some of the Tour's steepest mountains. It was the gutsiest ride I've ever seen, especially when you consider that testosterone has fairly minimal effect on performance.*

After he was popped, I watched Floyd's press conference, saw his half-hearted denials (when asked if he'd doped, Floyd hesitated and said, "I'll say no"). I felt how trapped Floyd was. I could see he was going down the same path I did. He'd fight the test, and he'd in all likelihood lose. Watching it unfold on my laptop, I wanted to reach through the computer screen and give him a hug. I wondered how Floyd—

---

* Landis later admitted to taking two BBs and microdosing EPO during the Tour, but maintained he had not taken testosterone.

independent, fearless Floyd—would take it.*

I couldn't spend too much time worrying about Floyd, however, because the fallout from the Puerto investigation was causing me problems of my own. It didn't take long for some of Ufe's calendars and materials to be released on the Internet. Most of it was in code, but one item that wasn't was a handwritten bill Ufe had faxed to Haven, including mention of Siberia, that showed we'd paid 31,200 euros and still owed 11,840 euros. Anyone could see the 2003 doping calendar Ufe had prepared for me, the dates matching my race schedule, along with his scribbled notations for injections and transfusions he recommended. I denied that I was Rider 4142 and said I was innocent, but anybody with a brain could make the connection.

Later, others would wonder why only my race calendar was released and not similar materials related to younger, active stars like Alberto Contador, who was rumored to be the client code-named A.C. (though Contador has always denied this). I don't have an answer for that, other than the obvious one: the sport is skilled at protecting its assets. Faced with yet another devastating scandal, it responded with a time-honored strategy: scapegoat a few, preserve the rest, and keep moving forward.

When I was linked to Puerto, I was officially toxic.

---

* After learning of his positive test, Landis said, he considered coming clean. After reflection and conversation with Armstrong, he decided to fight the charges. He wrote a book, *Positively False: The Real Story of How I Won the Tour de France*, and, through the Floyd Fairness Fund, raised several hundred thousand dollars to assist his legal challenge. "If you're going to lie, you've got to lie big," Landis said. "That's what Lance taught me."

None of the big teams were returning my phone calls, and I found myself right back where I'd started in 1994: a guy on the outside, searching for a team.

In November 2006, I signed a $200,000 one-year contract with a small Italian team called Tinkoff Credit Systems, owned by a Russian restaurant tycoon named Oleg Tinkoff. Tinkoff was a bit of a gambler who was smart enough to spot a niche: he decided to sign riders who'd been popped and whom other teams were avoiding: myself, Danilo Hondo, Jörg Jaksche (he tried to sign Ullrich, but Ullrich was still suspended).

The 2007 Tour of Italy, in May, was going to be my first big race back. Before the race, I showed exactly how much my suspension had changed my attitude: I got hold of some EPO from an Italian racing friend, and dialed myself up to some decent levels. I might have been a cheater, but I wasn't an idiot. With no BBs, I had zero chance at winning the race, of course; winning a stage would be victory enough.

The day before the race started, the UCI, in one of its patented "let's-pretend-to-clean-up-the-sport" moves, pressured the teams not to start any riders who were associated with the ongoing Operación Puerto investigation. Jörg Jaksche and I were booted from the Tour, Tinkoff stopped paying me, and I started looking for another team.

That fall I signed a $100,000 contract with Rock Racing, a new American team started by a charismatic fashion magnate named Michael Ball. Ball was out to create a team with a rock-and-roll vibe, and he knew that infamy can sell, if it's packaged right. Along with me, he signed fellow Puerto refugees Santiago Botero and Óscar Sevilla. With a roster like that, we knew we weren't going to get invited to the Tour de France. But we were good, and we had fun. In fact, we kind of relished being the bad boys of the sport; we grew our hair longer, we had cool uniforms, Ball threw big parties and drove fast cars. It felt good to let loose.

It was ironic. During my career, I'd looked like a Boy Scout and doped; now, in my comeback, I looked like a rock-and-roller and raced mostly clean, without Edgar. (I did take testosterone a couple of times.) Be assured: it wasn't some kind of moral stand. I'm sure that if somebody had offered me Edgar, I would have taken it, no questions asked. I knew the world hadn't changed—the guys at the top were still playing the game the same as they ever had, though with a bit more scrutiny from the testers. I just didn't have the connections anymore and besides, we were racing shorter races, mostly in the U.S., against lesser competition. I did find it gratifying that I could still get results riding on bread and water, just as I had when I was a neo-pro.

One thing that was less gratifying was the way some riders acted when I rejoined the peloton for bigger races like the Tour of California. I'd always had a lot of friends in the peloton; I'd always prided myself on the way I treated people. I didn't expect to be treated like a conquering hero, but I did expect riders to at least say hello, to be somewhat friendly. A few guys were great—I remember Chechu Rubiera was warm and welcoming. But on the whole, the peloton didn't exactly welcome me back.

One time early in my comeback, I was in a race with Jens Voigt. Jens is one of the best-liked guys in the peloton. He's funny, outgoing, and we'd always gotten along well. I was excited to see him, so I rode up next to him, expecting a chat. I saw him glance at me, then stare straight ahead. I wasn't sure what to do. We rode that way for a solid minute, inches apart.

Maybe he's kidding, I thought. *Maybe it's a joke, and he's about to crack a smile.*

Nope.

"Hey, Jens," I finally said, trying to sound cheerful. "How you doing today?"

He didn't look. "Just trying to follow the wheel in front of me," he said emotionlessly.

I waited, not quite able to absorb it. Then, shaking my head in sadness, I rode away. I tried not to take it personally. Maybe Jens was just afraid of being associated with me. Maybe I was an unwelcome reminder of what might happen to him if he got popped. Maybe it's just the way the brotherhood works. You're in or out. No in between.

Back home, Haven and I continued to drift apart. For much of 2007 I trained in Italy with Cecco, while Haven stayed in Boulder, earned her real-estate license, and got her career going again. When I was away, we didn't talk much, and when I returned, I was no picnic to live with, dealing with the stress of the comeback as well as my depression. Also, when you have to try to explain to your wife's parents why their last name was on a fax from a notorious Spanish doctor, that's tough. Our house in Sunshine Canyon began to feel like a museum of the hopes we no longer had. We were zombies, going through the motions, and at some point it became clear that it wasn't going to work anymore. By fall 2008 we had divorced. We kept it simple and cordial: one lawyer, everything split down the middle, no muss, no fuss, lots of good wishes for each other. It felt like we were climbing out of the wreckage, shaking hands, and heading our separate directions.

In early 2008 Rock Racing was invited to the Tour of California: a big race, a chance for me to show what I could do. Then, as at the Tour of Italy, organizers jerked the rug out from beneath us, excluding any riders tainted from Operación Puerto. It wasn't fair—I'd served my suspension, and should have been free to ride. Plus we had Botero and Sevilla, both of whom had flown thousands of miles to be there. We decided to stay with the team out of protest, hoping that other riders would speak up for us. But nobody did. They were afraid that they'd sully their images by supporting "known dopers."

I channeled my anger and won a couple of big races, the Tour of Qinghai Lake in China and, in August, the U.S. National Road Race Championship. It felt good to have some measure of redemption—especially in the latter race, when I beat my old roommate George Hincapie and a large crew of top American pros.

But the satisfaction was short-lived. Every victory was shadowed by a sense of how much had been lost, every interview echoed the story of my positive test, reminded me that there was no way to escape my past. The fact was, I was damaged goods, a thirty-seven-year-old bike racer with a tainted reputation, bouncing from race to race, with no wife, no home, no future prospects. I started drinking too much; my depression got worse.

In the fall of 2008, Lance surprised the world by announcing he was coming out of retirement and making a comeback. He said he was coming back to help raise cancer awareness, but to me the real reason was crystal clear: with all the scandals, his legacy was being battered, and he wanted back in the game, to take control of the story again. Why not? He could beat the tests, work hard, and play the old game. As ever, he had that old itch to raise the stakes. A big win, and everybody would shut up.*

As Lance was coming back, I was headed in the opposite direction. In early 2009 I tested positive again. I was trying to find a natural substitute for my depression meds, and in doing so tried an over-the-counter herbal antidepressant that contained DHEA, a banned substance which is not performance enhancing. I knew perfectly well that DHEA was banned, but I was desperate for help and I figured that the odds of my getting popped were remote. Of course, that was the one time in my career when the testers did their job—they caught me off guard (now that I was living alone, I didn't have the usual early-warning system).

---

* Though Armstrong had publicly cut ties with Ferrari in 2004 after the doctor was convicted by an Italian court for doping fraud and illegally acting as a pharmacist (the first conviction was later overturned on a statute of limitations argument, the second on appeal), the two kept in touch. Armstrong said the connection was purely personal, and that Ferrari no longer coached him. However, several Postal riders reported seeing Ferrari and Armstrong training together in Girona in 2005.

I think down deep I wanted to get caught. When I was called for testing at 6:30 a.m., I didn't even care enough to pee beforehand, which would've cleaned out my system and diluted my urine sample. When I was informed I'd tested positive, I felt an overpowering reflex to fight the test, to prove they were wrong (funny how strong habits are). But after talking to some friends, I had a moment of insight. I decided to try a strange new tactic: I'd tell people what really happened.

So I did. I called a press conference, took a deep breath, and laid out the facts. For the first time in my life, I talked openly about my depression. I talked about how I hadn't wanted to admit the condition because I was afraid people would see it as a weakness. I talked about my attempt to go off my prescription medication (which had recently been diminishing in its effectiveness, as happens with anti-depressants), and how I'd found the herbal antidepressant. I told them that yes, I'd taken the supplement, and yes, I'd known it contained DHEA.

I also told them that I was retiring, effective immediately. As I talked, I felt my heart lift: I didn't have to hire lawyers, I didn't have to strategize or pick my words or carry around secret knowledge. I could just tell what happened, just as it was. In the days afterward, I felt some part of me open up, like a fist that was starting to unclench.

I began reconnecting with family. The previous fall my mother had been diagnosed with breast cancer, and I started spending more time helping her with her recovery. I began to see a therapist in Boston, and the sessions were a huge help. He helped me start to pull back and look at life from a new point of view. I began to let go of some of the guilt I'd felt, to see just how crazy my life had been. I connected with old friends. Went to Red Sox games. Spent time with my parents, with my sister and brother and their families.

In January of 2010, I moved back to Boulder and started a small training business. I kept things simple: we didn't use a lot of computer-based training; instead, with the help of my friend Jim Capra, we outlined individual training programs and helped people toward their goals, whether it was to make the Olympic team or to lose fifty pounds. We got a few dozen clients, ranging from top prospects to newbies. I kept up the charity work with MS; my father and I continued organizing our yearly fund-raising ride called MS Global.

Best of all, I was dating a wonderful woman named Lindsay Dyan. Lindsay was beautiful, whip-smart, witty as hell, and had a spontaneity about her that I loved. We'd met in Italy during my comeback; we'd kept in touch and now we found ourselves arranging our schedules so we could be together. She was a true Bostonian, from a close-knit Italian family, earning her masters in international affairs and ethics from Suffolk University. She brought a lightness to my life that felt fresh and new, a sense that every day held new possibility. Just for fun, I once tried to capture Lindsay's personality on a Post-it note, and came up with three words: NUTTY. FUN. ALERT. And it's true. Once, she fell in love with a vintage 1979 Jeep Grand Wagoneer on eBay; the next thing I knew, we were flying to Texas to pick it up and drive it back to Boulder. We dubbed it the Green Machine, and we used it to explore the mountains around town. I think Lindsay thought of me like that truck: high mileage, a few dents, but worth taking a chance on.

This was going to be my new life. I tried to live under the radar. I didn't watch any of the Tour. I spent time with friends and took long runs in the mountains with Tanker, my new golden retriever, who was Tugboat's equal when it came to endless energy. I played indoor soccer, and I ran the business, and steered clear of Boulder's ultra-competitive bike-racer scene. I didn't really have a clear view of the future, except that I'd keep trying to have more good days, to move forward and be a normal person.

I thought that was the end of it. I thought all the drama with Lance was over and done with and buried. But as I was about to find out, the past wasn't dead. It wasn't even past.

Chapter 14

NOVITZKY'S BULLDOZER

A QUIET EVENING IN the middle of June 2010, and I was at home in Boulder. I was lying on my bed watching a cops-and-robbers movie, *The Bank Job*. Halfway through, my phone buzzed with a text.

> I'm Jeff Novitzky, an investigator with the FDA. I'd like to talk to you; please call me at this number.

My heart thumped. I'd heard the name, of course. Novitzky had put Barry Bonds on trial and put other dopers, including Olympic gold medalist Marion Jones, behind bars. He was often compared to Eliot Ness, the straight-arrow cop who attacked corruption during Prohibition, and he looked the part: tall, skinny, shaved head, with an intense gaze. I'd been expecting—and fearing—that he would be getting in touch with me.

It had started a few weeks earlier, when Floyd Landis dropped a bomb: an emailed confession to USA Cycling authorities, complete with dates, names, and highly specific details about Lance and the Postal team. Soon the story was beaming around the world, and Lance was standing outside his team bus at the Tour of California making the usual moves: (1) act unsurprised; (2) call Floyd bitter, and hint that he has psychological problems; and (3) quietly start hiring expensive lawyers. It was only when *New York Times* reporter Juliet Macur brought up Novitzky's name that Lance got nervous. "Why would . . . why would Jeff Novitzky have anything to do with what an athlete does in Europe?" he stammered.

Lance was right to be nervous. Within days, a grand jury was empaneled in Los Angeles under the control of federal prosecutor Doug Miller, who'd worked with Novitzky on the BALCO case. Witnesses were being subpoenaed to testify, and they had to tell the truth, or risk going to jail for perjury. In short, it was Lance's worst nightmare—a powerful, sharp-edged legal inquiry into how he had won the Tour de France.

It was poetic and maybe inevitable that it was Floyd who finally blew the whistle: the Mennonite kid, the one who was Lance's equal when it came to never-say-die toughness. What bothered Floyd wasn't the doping. What he hated—what his soul raged against—was unfairness. The abuse of power. The idea that Lance was purposely depriving Floyd of an opportunity to compete.

That's all Floyd had wanted, to compete. When his suspension had ended, Floyd had tried to earn his way back into the peloton. When Lance and the sport ignored him and vilified him, Floyd was left to scuffle alone for a series of small teams. Lance could easily have landed

Floyd a spot on his or another team; all it would have taken was a thirty-second phone call. The whole investigation might have been avoided if only Lance had been able to be a friend to Floyd; to reach out, to smooth things over. But you might as well have asked Lance to ride to the moon. To Lance, friendship was unthinkable. Floyd was the enemy, and enemies must be crushed, period. This approach works with most people. But not with a tough Mennonite kid who can quote the King James Bible from memory, especially Numbers 32:23: *Be sure your sin will find you out*. In April of 2010, Floyd contacted Travis Tygart, CEO of USADA, and began to tell him the truth about his time on the Postal team.

Novitzky had entered the situation months earlier. His involvement started after performance-enhancing drugs were found in the refrigerator of a rented apartment in Calabasas, California, that had been rented by a former Rock Racing rider named Kayle Leogrande. On discovering the stash, the landlord contacted the Food and Drug Administration, for which Novitzky had recently begun to work, and Novitzky got in touch with USADA's Tygart, with whom he had a long-standing relationship. All of which meant that when Floyd started talking to USADA, it wasn't long before he was also talking to Novitzky.

Floyd told the truth to Tygart and Novitzky, and apparently did his legal homework as well. The False Claims Act is a civil statute designed to protect the government against fraud by entitling whistleblowers to 15 to 30 percent of the recovered funds. Given that the U.S. Postal Service had paid Tailwind Sports (the

management company partly owned by Lance) more than
$30 million to sponsor the Postal team, the statute could
potentially apply—particularly if Tailwind was proven to
have violated anti-doping clauses in its contract by
running an organized doping program. According to
reports, Floyd filed a False Claims Act lawsuit against
Tailwind Sports after he started talking to USADA and
Novitzky. It was poetic: if Lance and Tailwind were
proven to have defrauded the government, Floyd might
be entitled to a biblical retribution.

Floyd's final decision was made in the weeks leading up
to May's Tour of California, the year's biggest domestic
race. Via email, he informed race director Andrew
Messick that he had been speaking with USADA about
his time on the Postal team. (Being Floyd, he even invited
Lance to attend his meetings with USADA.) When Floyd
saw that Lance and Messick were going to continue to
ostracize him, he wrote the confession emails to USA
Cycling, and the fuse was lit.

Essentially, Novitzky and Miller drove a bulldozer
into the bike-racing world. Before long everyone was
buzzing with fear and anticipation. Witnesses were being
contacted: Hincapie, Livingston, Kristin Armstrong,
Frankie and Betsy Andreu, Greg LeMond, and so on. I
heard Levi Leipheimer had received his subpoena at
customs when he returned from the Tour de France.
Armstrong's teammate Yaroslav Popovych was served his
subpoena in even more dramatic fashion: by agents in a
black Suburban, who waylaid him while he was visiting
Austin for an Armstrong cancer-awareness event that fall.

Then came the night Novitzky's bulldozer rumbled up

to my door, in the form of his text message. I put Novitzky in touch with my lawyer, Chris Manderson. When Novitzky asked Chris if I was willing to voluntarily cooperate with his investigation, I gave a firm no. The old logic applied: Why would I volunteer my testimony after denying it all for so long? Why would I risk ruining whatever was left of my reputation? I wanted to get on with my life, not go backward. A few days later, Novitzky responded with a subpoena. I was ordered to appear in a Los Angeles courtroom on July 21, 2010, at 9 a.m.

As July 21 approached, my anxiety level rose. I spent nights lying awake, trying to figure out what to do. At times I'd think, *Screw it, I'll keep lying, I'll risk perjury*. At other times, I'd plan to take the "I don't recall" approach like I'd seen corporate and government officials do on television. Meanwhile my lawyer was receiving a series of urgent calls from Lance's lawyers, who were offering me their services, for free. It was a classic Lance move. For six years, he gives me zero support. Now, when things get tough, he wants us on the same team again. No thanks.

The day before my grand jury appearance, I flew to Los Angeles to meet with Manderson and Brent Butler, one of his fellow attorneys who'd previously worked for a federal prosecutor. We sat down in a small conference room. They suggested it might be useful if I ran through some of my testimony. They started with the simplest question: *Tell us about your early days on the Postal team.*

A river of images and memories flooded into my mind. Meeting Lance at the Tour DuPont, Thom Weisel's gravelly voice, the white bags, the red eggs, Motoman and Ferrari and Ufe and Cecco. I took a deep breath and started from the beginning, as best I could. I saw Manderson and Butler go still. They sat back; they stopped asking questions, and just listened, their eyes fixed on me. It seemed like an hour, but when I looked up, four hours had passed.

It sounds strange, but I'd never told it like that, all of it, from beginning to end. Telling the truth after thirteen years didn't feel good—in fact, it hurt; my heart was racing like I was on a big climb. But even in that pain, I could sense that this was a step forward, that it was the right thing to do. I knew there was no going back. I understood what Floyd meant when he said that telling the truth made him feel clean, because now I felt clean, I felt new.

The next day I went to the federal courtroom in downtown Los Angeles with Manderson and Butler. We got there early, and Novitzky met us near the door. He was big (six-seven) and clean-looking, and his bald dome made him seem intimidating. But underneath he was more of a suburban jock dad: casual body language, easygoing voice, a leather bracelet beneath the white cuffs of his suit. Below his lip, he had a tiny soul patch. His manner set people at ease and made them feel safe: the word for him was "steady." I could see why Betsy Andreu called him Father Novitzky; he had a composure that you usually see only in priests and old people. We chatted for a while about basketball and the Red Sox. I couldn't help notice that Novitzky's command and confidence reminded me a little of Lance, with one difference: where Lance wielded his power like a cudgel, Novitzky carried his lightly.

Then, as the time for my questioning approached, Novitzky's easy smile was replaced by a businesslike demeanor that I would come to think of as his Investigator Face. He explained what was going to happen next: how I was going to be sworn in and interviewed by the prosecutor, Doug Miller. Novitzky didn't coach me or steer me in any way; he didn't talk about Lance or the investigation; in fact, he wasn't allowed in the grand jury room. He told me that my only job was to answer the questions as truthfully as I could. I took a breath and walked through the door with one thought: *No question is going to stop me.*

The questions began, and I answered them all in full. Instead of giving the minimum, I'd back up and tell them the background, fill in details. When they wanted me to point the finger at Lance, I always pointed it at myself first. I didn't just want to tell the facts. I wanted them to feel what it was like to be us. I wanted them to think about what they would have done in our situation. I wanted them to understand.

Miller did his best not to show any emotion, but occasionally I glanced over and his eyes were widening a bit. After four hours I was only partway through my story, but we'd reached the end of our court-allotted time; the grand jury was dismissed. I wanted to continue, however, and so did Miller. After talking to my lawyers, I decided to give the remainder of my testimony as a proffer, a standard legal arrangement for a cooperative witness which ensures my protection from any prosecution based on any admissions I might make—it's not immunity, exactly, but it's in the ballpark. I then gave three more hours of testimony in a conference room with Novitzky and my lawyers present, for a total of seven hours of testimony. When it was over, Novitzky and Miller thanked me. They tried to be objective and businesslike, but I could tell from their expressions they appreciated my honesty. They said they'd be in touch, and then I walked out the door. I was utterly exhausted, empty. But it felt good.

Even so, Lance never seemed far away. The morning after my testimony I was out on the street in front of the Mandersons' house in Orange County, teaching Chris's son how to ride a bike. I was running down the street, holding the bike, when a gray SUV drove past us, then braked suddenly to a stop. The window buzzed down, and I was astonished to see a familiar face: Stephanie McIlvain, the Oakley rep who'd been a friend of mine back in the Postal days. Stephanie had been in the Indiana hospital room when Lance made his alleged confession back in 1996. By pure coincidence, she lived near the Mandersons.

I was immediately wary, because I wasn't sure whose side Stephanie was on. In public, and under oath, she'd said that she hadn't heard Lance admit to drug use in that hospital room. But in private, she'd told a different story—she admitted that she'd indeed heard Lance's confession, and that he'd pressured her to keep quiet.*

---

* In the 2005 SCA Promotions hearing, McIlvain testified under oath that she had never heard Armstrong admit to doping. In a tape-recorded conversation recorded secretly the previous year by Greg LeMond, however, McIlvain says that she heard Armstrong confess in the hospital room. "So many people protect [Armstrong] that it's sickening," she said.

Stephanie seemed eager to talk. She asked for my phone number, and I gave it to her. An hour later, she started texting me, urging me to come over so we could visit some more. I begged off, saying I was busy. Then Stephanie sent another text. And another. Then another. Then she told me that another old friend, Toshi Corbett, who'd worked for the helmet company Giro, had come over and I should see him.

That made me even more wary. I presumed Toshi was firmly on Lance's side. I began to wonder if Stephanie and Toshi wanted me to come over so they could gather some intelligence and report it to Lance.

So I didn't text Stephanie back. I felt bad ignoring her, but I didn't want to take any risks; I didn't want Lance to know about my testimony. The next day, I headed back to Boulder, feeling like I was being watched.

I was now in the middle of things, smack between Novitzky and Lance, the hunter and the hunted. Not a day went by that I didn't think about both of them, picture their faces, or feel their presence in my life. They were playing chess, and I felt like one of the pieces.

In November 2010, Novitzky and his team traveled to Europe to gather evidence. They met at Interpol headquarters in Lyon with cycling and doping officials from

---

In September 2010, McIlvain testified for seven hours in front of the grand jury. Afterward, her attorney, Tom Bienert, said she had "a very emotional day" and that she had testified that she had never seen, or heard of, Armstrong using performance-enhancing drugs. Whether that was true or not remains to be seen; as *Bicycling* columnist Joe Lindsey sensibly pointed out, if it was a simple denial, why did it take seven hours?

France, Italy, Belgium, and Spain; the officials pledged they would help. To close the case, Novitzky was apparently seeking the original samples from the 1999 Tour, still frozen in a French laboratory. For me, it was surreal: Novitzky was hunting down that same EPO we'd used in 1999, the same molecules that had traveled across France on Motoman's motorcycle, the same batch of EPO that I'd shared. This made it clear to everyone that this wasn't an ordinary investigation, and Novitzky wasn't an ordinary investigator. "The Justice Department would not ordinarily spend [this] type of time and money without an extreme seriousness of purpose," said Matthew Rosengart, a former federal prosecutor.

Lance got the message. He also got out the checkbook and started loading up his team, hiring the guy known as the Master of Disaster, Mark Fabiani, who had defended President Bill Clinton during the Whitewater scandal and Goldman Sachs during its SEC fraud case. He also hired John Keker and Elliot Peters, trial lawyers who'd gone up against the government in major-league baseball drug cases, and they joined a team that already consisted of guys like Tim Herman, Bryan Daly, and Robert Luskin, who had defended President George W. Bush adviser Karl Rove in the Valerie Plame leak case. In short, Lance brought in the best lawyers money could buy.

This was his new Postal team, and it appeared that he was driving them hard, just like he'd pushed us. They issued statements wondering why the U.S. government should care about ten-year-old bike races in France, and complaining about the waste of taxpayer money. Meanwhile, Lance kept applying pressure through the media and his connections. He golfed with Bill Clinton and never missed an opportunity to meet a head of state, a celebrity, or a CEO. He invited influential members of the cycling media to his house for private conversations, and he kept sending upbeat tweets to his more than three million followers. The strategy was one that media advisers call "brazening it out": you simply keep going, pretending that the investigation doesn't exist.

Occasionally, though, Lance's old instincts got the better of him. When Novitzky traveled to Europe, Lance sent out a tweet: *Hey Jeff, como estan los hoteles de quatro estrellas y el classe de business in el aeroplano? Que mas necesitan?* (Translation: How are the four-star hotels and business class in the airplane? What more do you need?) Classic Lance: kinda funny but a couple notches too cocky, especially considering that Novitzky was flying coach, and staying in such inexpensive hotels that one of his fellow investigators slept in his suit rather than risk getting bedbugs.

The trickle kept coming. In January, Selena Roberts and David Epstein of *Sports Illustrated* did a major, well-sourced story on the investigation that uncovered some interesting new material, including:

- An account from Motorola teammate Stephen Swart of how Lance urged the team to begin taking EPO in 1995. Swart also recalled that Lance had a hematocrit of 54 or 56 on July 17, 1995, four days before he won a Tour de France stage.
- A 2003 incident in a St. Moritz airport, when

Lance and Floyd were unexpectedly searched by Swiss customs agents. (One of the benefits of private jets, the story noted, was the lack of stringent customs checks.) Inside a duffel bag, agents discovered a cache of syringes and drugs labeled in Spanish. After persuading the agents that the drugs were vitamins and the syringes were for vitamin injections, they were allowed to pass.

- Floyd's account of Ferrari relating his worries that steroids had given Lance testicular cancer in the first place.

- An account, from a source familiar with the government's investigation, that Lance had, in the late 1990s, gained access to a blood booster called HemAssist, a new drug which was in clinical trials at the time. "If somebody was going to design something better than EPO, this would be the ideal product," said Dr. Robert Przybelski, who was director of hemoglobin therapeutics at Baxter Healthcare, which developed the drug.

Via Twitter, Lance responded to the story in the usual way: first with a casual shrug (on his Twitter account, he wrote, "*that's it?*"), and then a shot of brazenness: "*Great to hear that @usada is investigating some of @si's claims. I look forward to being vindicated.*"

I checked in with Novitzky occasionally; he didn't tell me all that much—he was careful to stay professional in that way. But as the months passed, we got to be comfortable with each other. He was always warm and relaxed and helpful; we talked about more than the case. We talked about his daughter's volleyball tournaments, his own athletic career (he'd been a high jumper and had once cleared seven feet). He said "bullshit" a lot; he called me "dude."

You might think that Novitzky hated Lance, but whenever we talked about Lance, Novitzky became the cool professional; he never got emotional or offered his opinion on Lance's character, never called him a name or cursed. I know that Novitzky has sympathy for dopers in general. He'd met enough of us to realize that most of us aren't bad people; he certainly treated my situation with empathy. But did that empathy extend to Lance? I don't think so. When Lance's name came up, Novitzky was cold, factual, focused. I think he disliked what Lance represented: the idea that one person could use his power to flout the rules, lie to the world, make millions, and walk away scot-free.

In March, I was contacted by *60 Minutes* producers working on a major investigative piece on Armstrong. According to their sources, indictments were on the way soon; the producers said that my going on *60 Minutes* would be a good chance to tell my side of the story. After weeks of hesitation, I agreed to fly to California in mid-April and sit down with *60 Minutes* correspondent and CBS News anchorman Scott Pelley for an interview. Before I could do that, however, there was something I had to do first, something I'd been dreading: tell my mom the truth.

I'd told my dad earlier; I'd just blurted it out to him one night earlier in the year, when I'd been visiting home.

He didn't believe me at first—then, all at once, he did. He tried to keep his chin up in the best Hamilton tradition, but I could see the pain on his face; I felt like I'd stabbed him in the gut. After talking about it more—after hearing about the investigation and the coming indictments—he'd seen the logic; he'd understood, and he'd seen how much better I felt. Still, Dad had suggested we hold off telling Mom for a while, and I had agreed.

But now I couldn't hold off anymore; my interview was a few days away. The moment came during a family gathering at my parents' house in Marblehead. I was nervous, almost trembling, trying to pick the right time. It felt like that moment in a crash when you're still falling and there's nothing you can do to stop it. So I did what I did then: I shut my eyes and just got ready for impact. Toward the end of the party, everyone was eating chocolate cake, and there was a pause in conversation. I took a deep breath. Now.

I've got something I want to tell you guys. Something big.

Their first reaction was to smile—was Lindsay pregnant? Then they saw the expression on my face, and they froze.

Something I should have told you all a long time ago.

I think in their hearts they knew what was coming. They probably knew subconsciously all along. But it didn't make it any easier. The fact was, they'd all worked so hard for me all these years, defended me, loved me. Believed in me.

I started to tell them, and then I lost it when I looked at my Mom's eyes, which were filling up with tears. I took some deep breaths, looked away. I told it as quickly and plainly as I could. I told them about the investigation, and the trial, and how all the secrets were coming out. I told them that I needed to tell the truth for myself, for the sport. I told them that sometimes before you can go forward, you have to take a step back. I told them I had so much more to tell them, that I knew they couldn't really understand now, but that someday I hoped they would. Then my mom gave me a hug.

I felt the hug, and I realized: she'd never cared if I won the Tour or came in last. All she cared about was one question. She asked it now: "Are you okay?"

My smile showed her the answer. *I'm okay*.

A few days later I flew out to California. Being interviewed by *60 Minutes* is a combination of luxury and torture. You're taken to a five-star hotel, you sit in a cushy chair surrounded by super-nice production people who do their best to make you relaxed and comfortable, and then—*click!*—the lights come on, and they steadily begin peeling back your life layer by layer. Pelley asked all the tough questions, and I told him the truth as best I could. He was focused like a laser on Lance, of course, and I did my best to redirect him toward the bigger picture, to tell him that Lance didn't do much the rest of us weren't doing, to show him the world we were living in.

At one point, we were talking about my decision to dope back in 1997. I told Pelley how I had been so close to my goal of riding a Tour, how it had felt like an honor to be asked to dope by the team doctor, how I felt like my choice was to either quit or join. I asked Pelley: *What would you do?*

I'm glad I asked him that question, because I think everybody who wants to judge dopers should think about it, just for a second. You spend your life working to get to the brink of success, and then you are given a choice: either join in or quit and go home. What would you do?

Chapter 15

HIDE-AND-SEEK

60 MINUTES AIRED ITS REPORT on May 22, 2011. Along with my interview, the broadcast included details of George Hincapie's proffered testimony, in which he allegedly told investigators he had shared EPO with Lance. (George did not deny the report.) Frankie Andreu appeared, telling about the high speeds of the EPO-fueled peloton, saying, "If you weren't taking EPO, you weren't going to win." *60 Minutes* also gave details behind Lance's suspicious EPO test at the 2001 Tour of Switzerland, and the UCI-instigated meetings Lance and Johan had with the lab director that helped make the test disappear. Lance was offered the chance to come on air and tell his side; he refused. A few days before the broadcast, I gave my Olympic gold medal to USADA, until such time as they could decide where it belonged.

I watched the show in Marblehead with my family and Lindsay. My family was incredibly supportive, of course, but I had no idea how it was being seen by the larger world. People had spent years believing Lance; it was natural to be pissed at me for telling the hard truth. Back when Floyd spoke out, some people had showed up at races waving signs with pictures of a rat on them. Would that happen to me?

Over the following days, I could feel people eyeing me, recognizing me. While I waited in the ticket line at the Boston airport, a passenger walked up to me, shook my hand, and congratulated me for telling the truth. Then on the plane, someone from across the aisle passed me a note: *I appreciate your honesty. You did the right thing.* On Facebook, people left dozens and dozens of supportive messages. A few days later, my parents mailed me a two-inch-thick stack of emails and letters they'd received. Keeping to that Hamilton honesty, they didn't filter the letters. Some people attacked me, said I had to be lying because I'd lied before. But the overwhelming majority were positive. They used words like "courage" and "guts," words of which I didn't consider myself remotely worthy. But it felt good to read.

Lance and his team responded, too. Fabiani said I'd duped *60 Minutes* and accused me of "talking trash for cash," demanded a retraction from CBS (a demand that was soundly rejected), and sang the usual refrain about wasting taxpayer money. They also put together a website called Facts4Lance, on which they tried to attack my and Frankie's credibility (though not George's). But in all it was pretty weak stuff; in part because they didn't have many facts, and also because they failed to reserve the Facts4Lance Twitter name, which was quickly scooped up by friends of Floyd Landis, who then filled the feed with their unique brand of heckling. Before long, Facts4Lance sputtered and was shut down. I found myself a little surprised. I'd expected Lance to attack me personally. The quiet made me wonder: Was he giving up? Had he lost his desire to fight?

I should have known better.

Earlier that spring, I'd accepted an invitation from *Outside* magazine to attend a June 11 event in Aspen, Colorado. I was happy for a chance to promote my training business, and the chance to see some old friends. As the date approached, though, I grew nervous. I knew that Lance was spending a lot of time at his home in Aspen with his girlfriend, Anna Hansen. But just before the event, a friend checked Lance's schedule and told me he would be riding a 100-mile fund-raiser in Tennessee on June 11.

Good, I thought. *This way our paths won't cross.*

It was a beautiful day. I led an afternoon ride through the mountains with my colleague, Jim Capra. It was designed for intermediate-to-advanced riders, but we were joined by one ambitious beginner, a young woman named Kate Chrisman, who showed up with tennis shoes and an old bike with toeclips. She rode along, and though she was worried about slowing us down, she did great.

After returning from the ride, Jim and I hung out at the Hotel Sky with the rest of the crew, enjoying the evening sunshine. I ran into my high school roommate and Boulder neighbor Erich Kaiter. We didn't have any plans for dinner, but an outgoing friend of mine named Ian McLendon asked if we'd like to join him and a few other friends, and we said yes. By 8:15 there were a dozen of us in our party, and, it being Aspen, two of them were reality-television stars: Ryan Sutter and his wife, Trista, from *The Bachelorette* and *The Bachelor*, along with their two kids. Ian chose the restaurant, a little place called Cache Cache, which is French for Hide-and-Seek.

What none of us knew was that Cache Cache was Lance's favorite restaurant—his hangout. The moment we walked in, the co-owner, a woman named Jodi Larner, recognized me and phoned Lance to tell him I was there. Later, Larner tried to explain her call as a courtesy she gives to Aspen's divorced couples: if one is in the restaurant, she notifies the other to avoid an awkward encounter. However, her call had the exact opposite effect, because it turned out Lance had just returned to Aspen from Tennessee. Within moments of getting Larner's call, he was headed straight toward me.

Later, I thought about the moment when Lance received Larner's call. I'm sure Lance assumed I'd come to Cache Cache on purpose, and I was daring him to come down, and he responded the only way he knew how. But even so, I'm surprised that Lance would choose to get in his car and come to the restaurant. Because you don't have to be a lawyer to know that if you're the target of a major federal investigation, it's probably not a great idea to seek out contact with likely witnesses.

Unseen by us, Lance walked in with Anna Hansen, and took a seat on a stool on the left side of the large, crowded U-shaped bar with a few people he knew. He was perhaps thirty feet from our table, where he had a clear view of the back of my head as I joined in the eating, drinking, and laughing. Around ten, Ryan and Trista decided to head home and get their kids to bed. The rest of us were finishing our meals, debating whether we should go grab a drink somewhere else. Around 10:15, I got up to use the bathroom, which was on the opposite side of the bar from where Lance was sitting.

When I came out of the bathroom, I headed back to my table. Then, out of the corner of my eye, I saw someone in the bar area waving to me—Kate Chrisman, the woman from our ride. I decided to say hello, and I started threading my way through the crowd toward Kate.

As I passed the bar, I felt something press hard against my stomach, blocking me like a gate, not yielding a millimeter. At first I thought it was one of my friends joking around—it was too aggressive to be accidental, so I smiled and turned, expecting to see a friendly face.

It was Lance.

"Hey, *Tyler*," he said sarcastically. "How's it going?"

My heart jumped to my throat. My brain couldn't quite register what was happening. Lance didn't move his hand, kept it pushed hard against my midsection, relishing the moment. He could see I was stunned. I took a step back to create some distance.

"Hey, Lance," I said stupidly.

"So what are you doing tonight, dude?" he asked, his tone light, contemptuous.

"I'm, uh, just having some dinner with some friends," I managed. "How are you?"

Lance's eyes were shining, his cheeks were pink, a whiff of alcohol on his breath. He looked bigger, thicker through the middle; the lines on his face were deeper. I saw a blond woman sitting next to him; his girlfriend,

I figured, along with a few people who, by their approving expressions, appeared to be Lance's friends.

"Look, I'm really sorry about all this shit," I said.

Lance didn't seem to hear. He pointed at my chest. "How much did *60 Minutes* pay you?"

"Come on, Lance. They didn't—"

"How much did they pay you?" Lance repeated, his voice rising. It was the same slightly-too-loud voice he used to use on the Postal bus, the everybody-listen-to-me voice.

"You know they're not paying me, Lance," I said quietly.

"How much are they fucking paying you?"

"Come on, Lance. We both know they're not paying me." I fought to keep my voice level.

Lance's nostrils were in full flare; his face was getting redder and redder. Across the room, I saw Kate Chrisman watching with a concerned look on her face.* I felt this was spiraling out of control; I wanted to defuse it.

"Lance, I'm sorry," I said.

"What the fuck are you sorry for?"

"It's gotta be hard on you and your family," I said. "With all this going on."

Lance tried to look incredulous. "Dude, I have not lost one minute of sleep over this. I want to know how much they fucking paid you."

---

* Chrisman, who was seated about ten feet away, said, "I couldn't hear what [Armstrong and Hamilton] were saying, but you could tell it was very ugly, and very tense. Lance was leaning forward, being the aggressor, Tyler was sort of shrinking, as if he wanted to get away. I remember feeling kind of scared, realizing that Lance Armstrong is totally freaking out, right here."

I pointed to my left, toward the restaurant door.

"Why don't we go outside and we can talk, one on one," I said.

Lance made a dismissive *phffffff*. "Fuck that. That'll be more of a scene."

I looked to my right and spotted a small room off the bar. It was empty. I pointed. "Okay, if we're going to talk, let's go in there," I said.

Inside, I'm thinking, *Lance, you piece of shit. If you really want to do this, let's get away from your posse and really talk about the truth, man to man.* I gestured to the room again.

Lance lowered his voice. He pointed at me.

"When you're on the witness stand, we are going to fucking tear you apart," he said. "You are going to look like a fucking idiot."

I didn't say anything. Lance was on a roll now. "I'm going to make your life a living . . . fucking . . . hell."

I stood there, frozen. Later, a lawyer acquaintance told me that I would have been smart to mark the moment by saying in a loud voice, "Did everybody hear that? Lance Armstrong just threatened me." But I didn't think to do that, because part of me wasn't believing that he was so stupid as to threaten me in public, and the other part of me was daring him to keep coming, keep talking, mother-fucker, bring it on, give me your best shot. It was our old dynamic: he provokes, and I match him. *Still here, dude.*

Over Lance's right shoulder, a small round face of a black-haired fiftyish woman appeared: Jodi Larner, the co-owner of the restaurant. Since she'd caused this encounter by phoning Lance, she figured it was time for her to play a role. She leaned in and pointed her finger at my chest.

"You are no longer welcome in this restaurant," Larner said. "You will never set foot in this restaurant again for . . . the . . . rest . . . of . . . your . . . *life*!" She glanced at Lance, looking for his approval. He nodded; she looked as if she might die from sheer satisfaction.

My mind was churning. The realization was sinking in: I needed to document this encounter, so I asked Larner for her business card. I apologized if we'd caused a disturbance. I was trying hard to keep it civil. Then I turned to Lance.

"Look, if you want to continue this conversation, I'm gonna ask one of my friends to join us. He won't say a word."

"Fuck that," Lance said. "Nobody fucking cares."

Lance was done. He'd delivered his message, impressed his posse, and rattled me—mission accomplished. He wasn't going to cooperate with me, so there was no point in trying. I turned to walk back to my table. But before I did, I took one step to my left, toward where Lance's girlfriend, Anna, was sitting. She was facing the bar, her body slightly turned toward Lance, staring straight ahead. She looked sad, as if she wished this would all just go away.

"Hey, I'm truly sorry for all this," I said. Anna gave the slightest nod; I could tell that she heard me.

As I walked back to our table; my insides were shaking. My friend Jim later told me that I was as white as a ghost. When I told him what happened, Jim thought I was kidding. Then I told the rest of the table what had happened. We ate the rest of our meal, ordered coffee and dessert, and we didn't look toward the bar. I knew that Lance would not leave until we did; he would stay there all night if necessary. After all, he had to win. We stayed for forty-five minutes. Ian paid the bill, and then we headed out.

Nine days later I walked into a Denver federal building and gave my sworn account of the encounter to prosecutor Doug Miller and two federal investigators via teleconference. I told them what had happened, and gave them the names of the various witnesses at the bar. The investigators were interested. They had a lot of questions about who had initiated the contact, what Lance had said, and how he had said it. They said they'd be in touch.

As the weeks and months passed, I tried to act cool on the outside, but in truth I wanted the indictments to come. After the Cache Cache incident, I wanted people (my family, especially) to see the truth; to be vindicated. I'd been told by Novitzky that it would be fairly soon. But as the weeks and months passed, all was quiet.

It wasn't that nothing was happening—quite the opposite. The investigation was rolling along; Novitzky and Miller were flicking levers on the bulldozer, more witnesses were being called before the grand jury, more evidence was being uncovered. Their challenge, as I understood it, wasn't that there was too little potential evidence but that there was too much: testimony from teammates, team management, tax stuff, urine samples, possible money transfers to Ferrari, and so on. I couldn't imagine how long it would take (the Barry Bonds case, which was a simple case of perjury alone, had taken six years so far).

I got on with my life. In August, three months after the *60 Minutes* report aired, I did something I hadn't done in a long time: I attended a bike race as a spectator. The USA Pro Cycling Challenge came near Boulder, and many of the top American pros were there. It was strange to be on the other side of the looking glass.

I stood by the road and watched the peloton go by. I felt the breeze as they cruised past me. I saw how powerful they were, skinny as blades, their bodies humming through the air, almost like they were flying. I saw them after the race, looking completely destroyed. *I used to be like that*.

People recognized me, and most of them were nice. I must've signed thirty autographs; people told me they were proud of me for being honest. One father told me that he'd made his kids watch the *60 Minutes* interview four times. (I feel sorry for your kids, I joked.)

Often when I saw someone from the product side of the industry, things got strange. They would hesitate, stammer, and brush me off. Some were simply cold; they'd barely look me in the eye. I understood why. These people couldn't afford to piss Lance off. Their incomes depended on keeping the myth alive. But it didn't make it any easier. I was still an outcast; still a stranger in my own sport.

But the encounter that meant the most happened after the race, when I spotted Levi Leipheimer riding past me on his way to doping control. I said, "Hey Levi, Tyler!"

Levi recognized my voice, stopped, turned around. We

talked for two minutes. Levi knew the score: he'd been subpoenaed; he knew a lot of the things I knew, and I assumed he'd told the truth. We didn't talk about much on the surface, but just connecting with him felt great. He couldn't have been more friendly, asking a couple of times how I was doing, wishing me well. It felt good to know that, at least in Levi's eyes, our brotherhood was still strong.

Life went on, as we waited for the indictments to be announced. Lindsay and I, who were now engaged, decided to spend the fall in Boston as she finished up her master's degree. Tanker and I moved into her cool little apartment in Cambridge, within an hour's drive of my folks in Marblehead. It was great to be back on the old home turf. We could root for the Red Sox, see old friends, and spend time with both our families. There was just one nagging thing: an increasing feeling that we were being watched.

It was small things at first. We'd notice people watching us in the grocery store or on the street. One time there were two guys who sat in a tan Ford Astro van on the street in front of our apartment for several hours, then reappeared the following day in a different car. Some mail disappeared from our front hallway, including some tax forms.

More disturbing, our computers and phones started behaving strangely: we'd be reading our emails on Gmail and suddenly we would find ourselves signed out, as if someone else had signed in. We heard strange beeps on our phones. We'd send a text, and find that it had sent two copies, not one. We changed our passwords, and told ourselves it was nothing. But as time went by, it continued. If there were hackers, they had a sense of humor: we began to see pop-ups for the Lance Armstrong Foundation all over the place, even when we were on sites that were unrelated to anything that might be connected to Lance or the foundation. I shared my concerns that our phones had been hacked with my dad, who did his part by ending our telephone conversations with ". . . and by the way, fuck you, Lance."

After a few weeks of this, I phoned Novitzky to tell him about these incidents. He was utterly unsurprised; in fact, it sounded as if he had been expecting it. Novitzky said that similar things happened to all the witnesses in the Barry Bonds case. Hiring a private investigator to follow potential witnesses was apparently standard operating procedure by the defense in these cases: the more information they had on me, the easier they could attack my credibility in the trial. Novitzky promised he had our backs: if we ever felt threatened, we should get in touch right away. He gave me a special number to call in emergencies, twenty-four hours a day. His support was professional, but done in an easy, friendly way we appreciated. He even sent a smiley face at the end of one of his texts. Lindsay and I got a kick out of that—the big, tough government investigator, using emoticons.

Fall reminded me why Boston is my favorite city on earth. It's not just the colors; it's the feeling of life busting out at the seams, a feeling of something falling away and some new surprise getting ready to show itself. While

Lindsay spent her days studying, Tanker and I spent our days exploring. We met a neighborhood teenager named James, who attended a special-needs school. James and Tanker took to one another like wildfire, and James started coming by to take Tanker on walks.

Before long, James and I were going on bike rides, with Tanker running alongside. We rode up Heartbreak Hill, the famous ascent of the Boston Marathon, and James did great; he was strong and determined. When we got to the top, James was as stoked as if he'd just climbed Alpe d'Huez. I was, too.

I kept visiting Dr. Welch, the therapist, and enjoying our talks. As our time went on, I opened up more and more to him. As the weeks passed, I realized that I was experiencing a strange feeling. I felt strangely light, almost giddy. I'd find myself chatting with people I ran into, or just standing stock-still on the sidewalk with James and Tanker, enjoying the feeling of the sun on my skin. That's when I realized what the unfamiliar feeling was: I was happy. Genuinely, deeply happy.

Here's what I was learning: *secrets are poison*. They suck the life out of you, they steal your ability to live in the present, they build walls between you and the people you love. Now that I'd told the truth, I was tuning in to life again. I could talk to someone without having to worry or backtrack or figure out their motives, and it felt fantastic. I felt as if I were back in 1995, before all the bullshit started; back when I had that little house in Nederland, Colorado, just me and my dog and my bike and the big world.

Lindsay's place was filled with books—philosophy,

psychology, sociology. I started reading them, feeling a side of my brain stretch for the first time in a long time. We watched less television, drank a lot of tea, did yoga. One evening, when I bent over to pick something up, I felt something strange in my midsection—a small roll of fat, for the first time in years. I pinched it, and it felt good. Normal.

I sometimes thought about what would happen if Lance went to trial. I always figured that it'd come down to a trial—Lance didn't seem inclined to cop a plea. Knowing him, he'd keep raising the stakes rather than settle. And knowing Novitzky, he wouldn't let up either, and the whole thing would wind up in court. It figured to be a zoo; the biggest sports-crime trial ever. The media would have a field day; it would make the Bonds and Clemens trials look like traffic court. People would know the truth about our sport, and they could make up their own minds. They could forgive Lance, or they could hate him for lying, for abusing his power. But whatever they did, at least they'd have a chance to learn the truth and decide for themselves.

One afternoon, I was doing some business research on the Internet, looking at training websites. As happened sometimes, an ad with a photo of Lance popped up. Usually, seeing his face made me wince, and I'd click the window closed. But this time, for some reason, I found myself staring at his face, noticing that Lance had a big smile, a nice smile. It made me remember how he used to be, how good he was at making people laugh. Yes, Lance could be a bona fide jerk, a huge tool. But he's also got a heart in there, somewhere.

I studied the picture, trying to reconnect with that feeling, and to my surprise, I found myself feeling sorry for Lance. Not completely sorry—he deserved a lot of what was coming to him; he'd made his bed and now he would have to lie in it. But I was sorry in the largest sense, sorry for him as a person, because he was trapped, imprisoned by all the secrets and lies. I thought: *Lance would sooner die than admit it, but being forced to tell the truth might be the best thing that ever happened to him.*

Chapter 16

THE END-AROUND

LINDSAY AND I WERE MARRIED in Boston just before Thanksgiving 2011, and we started making plans to move back to Boulder. We weren't sure we were going to stay forever; I had so much history there, and the endurance-sports scene is so intense—only in Boulder are retired cyclists celebrities—that it sometimes felt stifling. But we'd try it out for a while; and Lindsay, as usual, was game. In late December, we hitched a trailer loaded with our few belongings to our SUV, and drove out of Boston, headed west. We traveled the southern route, through Charlottesville and Knoxville and Chattanooga, listening to Johnny Cash turned up full blast—"Monteagle Mountain," "Orange Blossom Special," "Folsom Prison Blues," "I Walk the Line." We watched the countryside roll past, opened our windows and felt the warm air on our skin. We felt like we were headed for the beginning of a brand-new life.

Lindsay and I arrived in Boulder in early January. We

moved into a bungalow on Mapleton Avenue, and I set about building the training business, introducing Lindsay to my friends, getting on with life. Or, I should say, I mostly did all those things. Part of my mind was always hovering apart, waiting for word of the indictments. Plus, we started getting that same eerie feeling that we were being followed: problems with the computer and phone, strange people sitting in cars outside our house. We ignored it as best we could, but after the Cache Cache incident, we felt vulnerable, especially with Lance a few hours away in Aspen. We tucked a baseball bat by the front door, just in case.

Friday, February 3, was a clear, bright day, and Lindsay and I were looking forward to a quiet weekend. We'd go for a hike with Tanker, meet up with some friends, and root for our New England Patriots against the New York Giants in the Super Bowl. We were coming back from the hike that afternoon when I got a text and saw a link to an article.

Feds Drop Armstrong Investigation

I felt like I was going to get sick to my stomach.

I tapped my phone with a trembling finger. It had to be a prank. Then I saw the other headlines; they matched. It was true. I typed out a tweet: *Are you F-ing kidding me?* Then I deleted it—better to stay cool until I found out more.

I drove home, feeling frantic. I flipped on the computer and read more stories. They all said the same thing: *Case closed, no explanation.* I called Novitzky; no answer. I read

Lance's short statement where he expressed his gratitude. I scanned the stories, which all said the same thing: a U.S. attorney named André Birotte Jr. had issued a press release at 4:45 p.m. Eastern Time, the ideal time to make sure it got as little attention as possible, a moment when sports journalists were focused on the Super Bowl.

> United States Attorney André Birotte Jr. today announced that his office is closing an investigation into allegations of federal criminal conduct by members and associates of a professional bicycle racing team owned in part by Lance Armstrong.
>
> The United States Attorney determined that a public announcement concerning the closing of the investigation was warranted by numerous reports about the investigation in media outlets around the world.

I read it three times. Then I walked into the kitchen and punched the refrigerator.

Lance had found a way. Lance's friends had found a way to beat Novitzky.

I didn't know what to do. I felt like my brain was short-circuiting, sparking and sputtering. It was like the worst bike crash, but without the satisfaction of the physical pain. I paced around our little house, trying to absorb what this meant—for me, for Lindsay, for my parents. Lindsay tried to comfort me with a hug, but I pulled away. Tanker started barking nervously. I kept circling, pacing the room like a trapped animal; after some hours of this, I fell on the couch and went into a dreamless sleep.

On Monday I talked to Novitzky. His voice was tight,

clipped. He did his best to stay professional, but I could feel the anger and frustration beneath.

"Over the weekend, I thought about leaving my job," Novitzky said.

"I thought about leaving the country," I said.

"Me too." Novitzky gave a rueful laugh.

All the news reports said the same thing: it had been an end-around, a surprise move: Birotte, a political appointee, had closed the investigation from the top, without consulting the prosecutor or the lead investigator. Birotte informed everyone in an email fifteen minutes before the press release was issued. Neither Doug Miller nor Novitzky was asked for his opinion on the evidence, on the solidity of the case they were building. Twenty months of investigation. Thousands of hours. Hundreds of pages of grand jury testimony and other evidence, tucked into a box, and filed away as if they never existed.*

---

* According to reports, sources within the FBI, the FDA, and the U.S. Postal Service were "shocked, surprised, and angered" at the unexplained closure. One source said there were "no weaknesses in the case." ESPN reported that prosecutors had prepared a written recommendation to indict Armstrong and others. A source close to the investigation said that Sheryl Crow had been subpoenaed a few weeks before the closure, and that she'd been a "star witness." Crow did not respond to interview requests.

Four possible factors behind Birotte's decision to close the case:

1. Birotte, who'd been appointed just 11 months before, wanted to protect President Obama from the potentially ugly spectacle of indicting an American hero during an election year.

2. Sports-doping cases were not going well for the government. Neither the Bonds nor the Clemens cases had as yet delivered any meaningful results, and had been closer to train wrecks than triumphs for the government. The Armstrong case was huge and expensive; why risk a loss?

The next couple of weeks were tough. Some days, I found it hard to get out of bed; other days I had bursts of anger and impatience that I had a hard time controlling. I wasn't easy to live with. Lindsay was incredibly patient in dealing with me. There was one bright side: overnight, Lindsay and I stopped getting the feeling that we were being watched. Our phones and computers stopped misbehaving. Mysterious people stopped parking outside our house or watching us in the grocery store.

I slept a lot. I stayed indoors; I avoided the coffee shops and restaurants on Pearl Street where bike racers hung out. I didn't shave. I didn't want to go online; I knew the Lance people would be seeing this as a triumph, and taking a victory lap. I saw my phone filling up with messages: from friends, from journalists seeking a comment. I ignored them, shut out the world. What could I possibly say?

Lance knew what to say. In an interview with *Men's*

3. Birotte was wary of the cancer lobby. A controversy had recently erupted when the Susan G. Komen Foundation withdrew $700,000 in funding for Planned Parenthood for what appeared to be pressure from the political right (which opposed Planned Parenthood's support of abortions). On Friday, February 3, the same day the case was dropped, the Lance Armstrong Foundation donated $100,000 to Planned Parenthood to fill the funding gap, providing a clear signal of the LAF's support of the Obama administration's stance on reproductive rights, as well as a connection to the millions of women who objected to the Komen Foundation's decision.

4. Birotte may have received the results of an internal leak investigation, and had decided those results would potentially embarrass the Department of Justice, if it showed government employees leaking to the media.

While some are inclined toward conspiracy theories, it makes more sense that Birotte made a political judgment that the risks of the criminal prosecution outweighed the rewards.

Journal, he talked about his relief at the closure, and said that he was through fighting. "In my mind, I'm truly done," Lance said, mentioning he would not fight if USADA attempted to strip him of one or more Tour titles. "It doesn't matter anymore. I don't run around bragging, feeling like I have to be a seven-time Tour de France champion. I worked hard for those, I won seven times, and that's great. But it's over."

Lance underlined that point in an interview with former San Francisco mayor Gavin Newsom. "If somebody wants to walk up and say, 'You know, I think you cheated to win the Tour de France seven times,' I would literally go, all right. Is there anything else? Because I'm not going to waste any more of *my* time talking about it, and you shouldn't waste *your* time talking about it. Let's move on."

I read his words with mixed emotions. Part of me had sympathy for Lance. I never wanted him to go to jail. I never thought of him as a criminal. But at the same time I did want—I do want—the truth to come out. That's what was so devastating: the sense of futility, the sense that all of it—my testimony, Novitzky's work, the risk I and others had taken by speaking out—had come to nothing.

When I did go out again, Boulder was feeling smaller and smaller. Every time we walked into a coffee shop I would get funny looks, or I'd see a yellow wristband, or see some guys in bike jerseys that said DOPERS SUCK. I was feeling suffocated, and Lindsay wasn't enjoying living inside of my checkered past.

We decided to leave Boulder. We'd been thinking about the idea for a while, and now it seemed more attractive than ever. We needed to start somewhere fresh. Somewhere where we had no past, no connections, no history dragging us down; somewhere we could maybe start a family. We set our sights on Missoula, Montana. Lindsay had an uncle who worked as a fly-fishing outfitter in Montana; she'd always dreamed of living there. She found a quote in *A River Runs Through It*, wrote it out in black marker on a big piece of paper, and stuck it to the refrigerator. *The world is full of bastards, the number increasing rapidly the further one gets from Missoula, Montana.*

That settled it. We would drive out, leave all this behind. Fresh start. Clean break. Goodbye, cycling; goodbye, Novitzky; goodbye, Lance.

In spring 2012 Lindsay and I moved to Missoula. We loaded up a rented U-Haul with our stuff, and we headed northwest like a couple of old-time pioneers, with Tanker riding shotgun. We rented a modest bungalow within a bike ride of downtown Missoula with a big yard for Tanks, a spare bedroom for our training-business home office, and plenty of squirrels to chase (not to mention the occasional grizzly).

Right away, life felt different. Lighter, more spontaneous, slower. We started taking time to enjoy the simple things: eggs Benedict on a random Tuesday, an early-morning hike, a road trip to Glacier National Park, a glass of wine as we watched the sun set in the Bitterroots. Lindsay and I would occasionally look at each other and just crack up at the craziness of the whole thing: we're living in Montana!

The world works in strange ways. I know that old saying that when God closes a door He opens a window. I think that saying is really talking about the resilience of truth. I've come to learn that truth is a living thing. It has a force inside it, an inner springiness. The truth can't be denied or locked away, because when that happens, the pressure builds. When a door gets closed, the truth seeks a window, and blows the glass clean out.

Around the time that we moved, my cell phone started to ring. The caller ID showed that the calls were coming from Washington, D.C., and Colorado Springs, headquarters of USADA. I ignored them at first, partly because I was exhausted from all this, and partly because I had a good idea what they wanted.

I'd heard that the Department of Justice's civil division in Washington had joined Floyd's case and wanted to find out if Lance and the Postal team owners had defrauded the government by falsely representing the team as clean. The DOJ investigators were assisted by the fact that civil cases are held to a different standard of proof from criminal cases: instead of "beyond a reasonable doubt," it's a "preponderance of evidence."

USADA was pursuing its own case. Unlike civil and criminal prosecutors, USADA didn't concern itself with laws, only with the rules of the sport. Travis Tygart, the CEO of USADA, had been aware of the federal investigation from the start, participating in some meetings and providing Novitzky and Miller with background information. While neither USADA nor the Justice Department's civil division would have access to the grand jury testimony, both would possibly have access to the proffers and the other materials the criminal investigation had produced.

In short, it was becoming clear that the bulldozer Novitzky had started was still running. My phone kept ringing, and with each ring the message was louder: the game was still on. USADA and the DOJ wanted to know, would I be willing to cooperate? Would I go under oath and testify?

I thought about it for a while. Then I called them back and told them yes, absolutely. I know it would have been easier to let it all go, to simply move on. But I couldn't do that. I'd started this race, and I was going to finish it.

In April, in separate interviews over two days, I told USADA and DOJ investigators what I remembered from my years with Postal and Lance. I gave them everything as precisely and completely as I could. I told the truth, the whole truth, and nothing but the truth.

I wasn't the only one. USADA investigators conducted similar interviews with nine other former Armstrong teammates, with similar results. Every Postal rider USADA contacted agreed to speak openly and honestly. USADA did not tell me who the other teammates were, but I could make a guess. All of us, together again, just like the old days in Nice and Girona. It was a strange feeling, talking to the investigators and knowing that the other guys were telling their stories as well. I found myself remembering those old days—back when we started out, those days in the Dee-Luxe Apartment in the Sky, that moment of innocence before all this craziness started. I wondered if they were feeling it too.

On June 12, 2012, USADA delivered: a simply worded

fifteen-page letter charging Lance, Pedro Celaya, Johan Bruyneel, Luis del Moral, Pepe Martí, and Michele Ferrari with anti-doping rule violations, alleging that they had conducted a conspiracy to dope "in order to advance their athletic and sporting achievements, financial wellbeing, and status of the teams and their riders." Lance was charged with use, possession, trafficking, administration, assisting, and covering up. USADA also said that data from blood collected from Lance during 2009 and 2010 was "fully consistent" with blood manipulation. Furthermore, Lance was immediately banned from participating in triathlon, a sport he'd returned to after his retirement.

The USADA charges changed everything. While Lance might've accepted losing one or two Tour titles, he clearly wasn't prepared to lose all seven, plus his future in triathlon. Lance's "I'm not gonna fight" stance shifted 180 degrees. His lawyers cranked up the attack machine and aimed it at USADA, attempting to paint it as bitter, vengeful, smug, irrational, etc. Via Twitter and his lawyers, Lance called the process "unconstitutional," complained about access to evidence, and issued what might rank as one of the most ironic tweets of all time: *It's time to play by the rules.*

While Lance has a considerable advantage in legal and PR firepower, he also had a disadvantage: USADA is not a court of law, and so is concerned only with the simple question of whether Lance and the others broke the rules of the sport. Instead of a federal trial, Lance would face an arbitration hearing; instead of being protected by a legal standard of "beyond a reasonable doubt," he would face the much lower standard of "comfortable satisfaction of the hearing panel."*

At this writing, the outcome is far from certain, but it's safe to say it's not going to be pretty. I'm sure Lance is going to do everything he can to attack my credibility, and that of his other teammates who are telling the truth. Lance provided a preview of his strategy on the day the USADA charges became official, when he leaked the identity of a previously anonymous USADA Review Board member, along with that member's recent arrest on a misdemeanor charge of indecent exposure. *The Wall Street Journal* reported that Livestrong sent a lobbyist to visit U.S. Rep. Jose Serrano (D., NY), who sits on the House Appropriations Committee, in order to talk about USADA and its pursuit of Armstrong. I can see why Lance is using this strategy—after all, it's worked in the past, and at this point he doesn't have many other options. And perhaps it will work again; perhaps the public will keep wanting to believe him; or perhaps they'll simply get tired of this and wish it would all go away.

One thing's for sure, though: the truth will keep coming out. More former racers will step forward as they

---

* If he loses his titles or is sanctioned for doping, Armstrong faces the possibility that other parties could take action against him. SCA Promotions, which had unsuccessfully battled Armstrong in 2005 over its obligation to pay $5 million in bonuses for winning the 2004 Tour de France, said it was planning to investigate the possibility of suing to recover its money. "We basically told him that we will be monitoring the case and that we're going after our money if he is stripped of the title," Jeffrey Tillotson, an SCA lawyer, told *The New York Times*. "They responded: 'Tough bones, it's not happening. I never cheated.' It was just the usual Lance: I'm 100 percent right, and you're 100 percent wrong."

get older, as they realize that it doesn't make sense to keep living a lie. They'll experience how good it feels to be honest; they'll realize it's okay to be open and let people look at all the facts, and decide for themselves. In the meantime, I'm going to keep telling my story—both in big ways, like this book, but also in my daily life.

Just before we moved to Montana, I was riding through Boulder with my friend Pat Brown. I was wearing jeans and sneakers, riding my town bike, a heavy, beat-up cruiser with upright handlebars and fat tires. Pat and I were waiting at a streetlight when two riders in dark Lycra cruised past us on thousand-dollar racing bikes. They must've recognized me, because one of them turned and gave me a long, meaningful look as he passed. As he rode past I could read the words on his jersey, written in big white letters: DOPERS SUCK. I felt the old adrenaline surge. Everything in my mind concentrated into a simple urge: I wanted to catch that guy.

Stay on my wheel, I told Pat, and I took off after them. It wasn't a fair fight: they had a hundred-yard head start on us, and they were going hard, and I was on a heavy old bike that must've weighed thirty pounds. It must've looked pretty funny: me, going like hell in my tennis shoes and fat tires, pounding along after them like a steam engine. They looked back a couple times; they knew we were there. But they couldn't get away. Over a mile or so, I reeled them in.

We caught them at a red light, and I coasted up close to them, then closer. I put my fat front tire right between their expensive bikes. They looked back, and I looked at them; I could see in their eyes they were a little bit scared.

Then I reached out and took the DOPERS SUCK guy's hand, and shook it. I gave him a friendly smile.

"Hey, I'm an ex-doper," I said. "But I don't suck. Have a good ride, guys."

They rode off, and Pat and I rode home, and my heart was full of happiness. Because, I realized, that's my story. Not a shiny, pretty myth about superheroes who win every time, but a human truth about one normal guy who tried to compete in a messed-up world and did his best; who made big mistakes and survived. That's the story I want to tell, and keep telling, partly because it will help the sport move forward, and partly because it helps me move forward.

I want to tell it to people who think that dopers are bad, irredeemable people. I want to tell it so people might focus their energy on the real challenge: creating a culture that tips people away from doping. I want to tell it because now I *need* to tell it, in order to survive.

Before we left for Montana, I had to deal with one final chore. Nine chores, actually: big plastic totes that I kept in the garage, which contained my past, in the form of photos, files, letters, race numbers, trophies, magazines, T-shirts. I'm a bit of a hoarder, and this was pretty much everything I'd ever gotten in my career (I even kept a matchbook from a French hotel). As I went through the containers, I was startled to see how much was contained inside.

I pulled out the artifacts: My race number, #42, and a course map from my first big race, back at the 1994 Tour DuPont, the day I broke through. T-shirts from the 2003 parade in Marblehead that said TYLER IS OUR HERO.

A shiny orange Wheaties box with Lance on the front in his yellow jersey. Baseball-type cards with our pictures on them, with all of us looking like superheroes. Wrinkled old race numbers, the ones that were pinned to my jersey. A big shoebox full of letters from fans, condolence letters about Tugboat, letters from MS patients telling me their stories.

Most of all, photos. Faces. Kevin's wild grin, Frankie's flinty, commanding gaze. Eki lifting a glass of champagne, his face cracking with an unlikely Russian grin. George and I, arm in arm, having a beer after the Tour, Christian's sly grin. The whole team standing together in the sunshine on the Champs-Élysées. My parents, standing proudly on the side of the road with a sign that says ALLEZ TYLER.

I thought I would hate looking through that stuff. I thought I would wince and want to bury it. And I was right—it did hurt, it hurt a lot. But I kept looking, pushing through, until I came to the simple truth: *All this stuff is my life*. All this crazy, messy, amazing, terrible, real stuff, that's my life.

I'm happy to see my sport cleaning itself up over the past few years. It's far from 100 percent clean—I don't think that's possible, as long as you're dealing with human beings who want to win—but it's significantly better, and slower. The winning time up Alpe d'Huez in the 2011 Tour was 41:21; back in 2001, a rider with that time would have finished 40th.* The improvement is mostly

---

* The UCI's internal testing numbers reflect this change. In 2001, 13 percent of riders were classified as having abnormally high or low levels of reticulocytes, or newly formed red blood cells (signs of EPO use and/or transfusion). By 2011, that number had dropped to 2 percent.

due to better testing, better enforcement, and the "biological passport" program where riders' blood values are more closely monitored. There's still no test for BBs, and if you believe the rumors (I do), riders who are determined to dope are resorting to smaller, less effective BBs.

Overall, though, things are moving in the right direction. You don't see whole teams dominate entire races as often as they used to. What's more, individual riders are having ups and downs; you can see that big efforts carry costs, exactly as they should. I like that kind of racing partly because it's more exciting, but mostly because I think it's honest. After all, it's the humanity we love in these races. Every day brings risks and rewards. You might win. You might lose. That's the point.

Now I spend my time training people, helping them on the journey, seeing their hard work pay off. Whether they are Olympic-level athletes or regular folks who want to lose a few pounds, I treat them the same. Along the way, I try to tell them a bit of my story, try to tell them what I've learned: that the person who finishes toward the back is often more courageous than the one who wins. I feel like I'm returning to my early days on the bike, to the person I used to be. I'm excited about the second half of my life.

One last story. It happened the night before the *60 Minutes* interview in Southern California. I was hanging out on the balcony restaurant of the hotel when some guests approached me, wanting to chat. They were huge bike-racing fans; they watched the Tour fervently every year. They knew all about my career, they had my poster on their wall, and they said they supported me, which I appreciated. Of course, they had zero idea that in a few hours I was going on *60 Minutes* and would be telling the truth to the world. Then one of the guests, a fit, forty-something guy named Joe, spoke up.

"Could you stay right there for one minute?" Joe asked. "There's someone I really want you to meet."

Joe left and shortly returned accompanied by a dark-haired boy in a Cub Scout shirt, obviously his son. The boy, who was about ten, stood tall and proud; his sleeve was decorated with merit badges.

"Hi, I'm Tyler," I said, shaking the boy's hand.

"My name's Lance," the kid said.

I must have looked bewildered. Joe touched me on the arm. "He was born in 2001," he said helpfully.

"Oh," I said, still absorbing the name, still staring at this kid who's looking at me like he knows something's up. I have no idea what to say or do, except to put my hand on the kid's shoulder and give him a smile. He smiled back.

We made some small talk, and all the while I'm feeling like shit. I'm thinking, I'm sorry, kid. I'm sorry that in a few hours, I will be hurting you and your family, busting up the nice feelings you've got for your name. I'm sorry, but the truth is the truth. I hope you can understand.

We talked. Young Lance and I shot the breeze about the Scouts, merit badges, pelicans, astronomy. The kid knew his constellations, and he showed me some; he knew how far away they were, how many years it took for the light to reach us. As we talked, I found myself comforted by this kid. I liked the methodical way he thought about stuff, figuring it out, and the role his father had in his life, guiding him. He was strong and smart; he was going to be okay.

I thought I would leave young Lance with a word of wisdom to tuck in his pocket for later, when all this came out, so he might understand. But of course when the time for goodbyes came, my mind was a blank; I couldn't think of anything. Only later did it come to me what I wanted to tell him, the same thing my parents told me so long ago.

The truth really will set you free.

Where Are They Now?

FRANKIE ANDREU: Works as director of Kenda/5-Hour Energy, a U.S.-based team, and also as a video commentator on the Tour de France for Bicycling.com. Resides with his wife, Betsy, and their three sons in Dearborn, Michigan.

JOHAN BRUYNEEL: Denied the USADA doping charges and chose to have his case arbitrated be-fore USADA's panel; his case will likely be heard in October/November 2012. Pending the result, Bruyneel took a voluntary suspension from his duties as director of RadioShack Nissan Trek.

DR. LUIGI CECCHINI: Lives in Lucca, Italy, where he still trains professional cyclists.

DR. PEDRO CELAYA: Denied the USADA doping charges, and has chosen to have his case arbitrated before USADA's panel; his case will likely be heard, along with Bruyneel's, in October/November 2012.

DR. LUIS DEL MORAL: Chose not to contest USADA's doping charges, and received a lifetime ban from cycling and any other sport governed by the World Anti-Doping Agency code.

DR. MICHELE FERRARI: Chose not to contest USADA's doping charges, and received a lifetime ban from cycling and any other sport governed by the World Anti-Doping Agency code (adding to the lifetime ban preventing him from working with Italian cyclists that he received in 2002).

In April 2011, *La Gazzetta dello Sport* reported that investigators had uncovered a network of money transfers organized by Ferrari valued at 15 million euros. Ferrari remains under investigation.

DR. EUFEMIANO FUENTES: In December 2010, Fuentes was arrested and charged with organizing a doping organization involving track athletes and mountain bikers. Police seized EPO, steroids, hormones, and blood-transfusion equipment, along with an assortment of blood bags. The case was later dismissed when the telephone taps and searches used to obtain evidence were ruled invalid. Fuentes maintains his medical practice near his home in Las Palmas, on the Spanish island of Gran Canaria.

GEORGE HINCAPIE: Retired from the sport after riding in his record 17th Tour de France in 2012 for BMC Racing Team. He lives in Greenville, South Carolina, with his wife, Melanie, and their two children.

BARTY JEMISON: Lives with his wife, Jill, in Girona, Spain, where they run Jemison Cycling Tours.

BOBBY JULICH: Retired from racing in 2008, and now works as an assistant director for Team Sky.

FLOYD LANDIS: According to published reports, Landis is the plaintiff in the ongoing civil case against Armstrong and the U.S. Postal Service team ownership. He lives in Southern California.

KEVIN LIVINGSTON: Owns and runs the Pedal Hard Training Center, located on the lower level of Mellow Johnny's, the Austin, Texas, bike shop owned by Armstrong. He lives with his wife, Becky, in Austin.

PEPE MARTÍ: Denied USADA's doping charges, and has chosen to have his case arbitrated before USADA's panel; his case will likely be heard, along with Bruyneel's and Celaya's, in October/November 2012.

SCOTT MERCIER: Works as an investment advisor in Grand Junction, Colorado.

HAVEN PARCHINSKI: Lives in Park City, Utah, where she works in property management.

BJARNE RIIS: After years of denying that he'd doped, Riis chose to confess after a former Telekom soigneur named Jef D'Hont authored a book, *Memories of a Soigneur*. According to the book, Riis won the 1996 Tour de France while taking 4,000 units of EPO every other day, plus two units of human growth hormone, and his hematocrit during the 1996 Tour registered as high as 64.

Riis held a press conference in May 2007, and admitted to taking EPO, cortisone, and growth hormones between 1992 and 1998. "I apologize," he said. "Still, I hope it led to some great experiences for you. I did my best." Riis went on to discuss his doping past in his autobiography, *Riis: Stages of Light and Dark* (Vision Sports Publishing, 2012). He is currently the director and a part-owner of cycling's Team SaxoBank-Tinkoff Bank.

JAN ULLRICH: After his 2006 bust for doping, Ullrich proclaimed his innocence and entered a long legal fight. In 2008 Ullrich agreed to an out-of-court settlement with German prosecutors in which they dropped fraud charges in exchange for an undisclosed six-figure fine. In 2012, the Court of Arbitration for Sport banned Ullrich from cycling for two years and stripped his results from May 2005 onward.

In a June 2012 statement, Ullrich admitted he'd worked with Fuentes, expressed his regret, and said he wished he had been more honest when his case began. He now makes his living running a cycling camp and promoting Alpecin, an anti-hair-loss shampoo with the tagline "Doping for Hair."

CHRISTIAN VANDE VELDE: Rides for the Garmin-Sharp team and lives in Girona, Spain, and Chicago, Illinois, with his wife, Leah, and their two children.

JONATHAN VAUGHTERS: Works as director of the Garmin-Sharp cycling team, and serves as president of the AIGCP (Association International des Groupes Cyclistes Professionels, professional cycling's teams organization).

HEIN VERBRUGGEN: Served as president of the UCI until 2005, when he became chairman of the Coordination Commission for the Beijing Olympics. In 2008, a BBC investigation questioned whether the UCI had accepted $3 million in unethical payments from Japanese race organizers; Verbruggen denied any wrongdoing.

THOMAS WEISEL: Lives in San Francisco with his fourth wife, and is no longer involved in professional cycling. In 2010, Weisel's company, Thomas Weisel Partners, was charged with securities fraud for illegally manipulating clients' accounts in order to secure large bonuses for its executives. In 2011, a regulatory panel ruled largely in TWP's favor, fining the company $200,000 and reprimanding it for its "egregious" failure to oversee its fixed-income desk.

Afterword

IN THE LAST FEW MONTHS, I've been thinking a lot about avalanches.

In Montana, where Lindsay and I live, you can sometimes see them in the mountains outside our windows, or when we're out skiing. But I also see them in my dreams at night. I think about them because until the moment they happen, avalanches are invisible. The world looks peaceful and balanced. Then—no one can predict when—one more snowflake falls, or the temperature rises half a degree, and the whole world starts to shift.

Dan and I had finished writing *The Secret Race* on August 15th, 2012, and the final manuscript was sent off to the printer, being turned into books. The publisher's lawyers were on high alert, fully expecting the usual Armstrong response: lawsuits, intimidation, threats, attacks in the media, and who knew what else. At the time, it looked like we might be in for a long, drawn-out fight. Lance was in his familiar spot, backed into corner, doing all he could to stop the USADA process. He had filed a lawsuit in Texas federal court, and enlisted powerful allies—most prominently Pat McQuaid, president of the UCI—to challenge USADA's right to bring its case. It seemed to be working, too: McQuaid was operating as if he were a member of Lance's legal team, writing letters that echoed Lance's talking points: *groundless charges . . . unfair . . . USADA has no jurisdiction.* Livestrong lobbyists made the same case in Congress, which held the purse strings on USADA's funding.

As Lindsay and I watched it all unfold from our Missoula living room, the pattern felt depressingly familiar: Lance and his all-star team of lawyers pushing all the right buttons, controlling the story. There was little reason to believe things wouldn't work just as they always had. After all, just six months before, U.S. Attorney André Birotte had swooped in to pull the plug on the federal criminal investigation without warning—why wouldn't something similar happen now?

But on August 20, a no-nonsense federal judge in Texas named Sam Sparks put a stop to all the maneuverings. He ruled against Lance's lawsuit, writing that Lance's protests about USADA's process were "without merit" and that the agency's rules were "sufficiently robust" to protect Lance's constitutional rights.

Like most, I figured this meant that Lance had no other option than to fight USADA in an arbitration hearing, just as I had done when I was busted for doping in 2004. I figured this meant we were in for a battle of the titans: Armstrong vs. Travis Tygart, with me and the other riders called forward one by one to testify before the three-person panel, and to be cross-examined by Lance's lawyers. We were wrong.

Three days later, Lance surprised the world by announcing that he was folding his tent; he would forgo a hearing and accept USADA's charges, while still denying that he'd doped. In a written statement, he called the process a "charade" and said he was "finished with this nonsense." "Today I turn the page," he wrote. "I will no longer address the issue."

In retrospect, it was classic Lance: a surprise retreat designed to shift the battlefield, distract the public, and attempt to keep the evidence out of view. USADA and Travis Tygart, however, did not turn the page. Instead, they lobbed a tersely worded hand grenade of an announcement: Lance would be immediately stripped of his seven Tour de France titles and banned for life from participating in any sport that followed the rules of the World Anti-Doping Agency, including triathlon.

I remember reading that and thinking: *Holy shit*.

I'd imagined USADA would take some of his Tour titles. I'd imagined that they might ban him for a few years. But this? This was the nuclear option: USADA was photoshopping Lance out of cycling history, and removing his path to a sporting future forever. If Lance had been gambling that Tygart would back down, he'd made a serious miscalculation.[*]

---

[*] Armstrong had met with Tygart twice during the investigation, and been given a chance to make a deal: cooperate and confess, and you can keep five titles and continue your triathlon career after a brief suspension. But Armstrong said no to Tygart's offer, and followed his old pattern: deny and attack. [Footnote continues overleaf.]

The more I reflected on USADA's decision, the more it made sense. Tygart may have looked like a coolheaded lawyer, but beneath he was a passionate advocate for the rights of the clean athlete, and the importance of changing cycling's win-at-all-costs culture. To let Armstrong walk away with anything less than the required penalty would be a signal that nothing had changed, that you could cheat your way to the top. To him, the Armstrong case was about the simplest idea: everyone should follow the same rules, period.*

The world reacted with amazement. We'd all become accustomed to the spectacle of high-profile athletes wriggling free of doping charges. But now Lance, the guy who'd denied harder than anyone, had accepted the severest punishment—the athletic equivalent of a death sentence—with barely a peep. In the public's mind, the question was, why? What truth was Lance so afraid of, that he would lose all his titles and accept a lifetime ban rather than face his accusers in an arbitration hearing? It was a remarkable moment, a silence before the storm. People wanted concrete answers, and nobody – not

---

Later, during his Oprah Winfrey interview, Armstrong reflected on his decision, saying, "Then [USADA] came to me and said, 'OK, what are you going to do?' To go back to that moment, I would say, 'Guys, give me three days.' I'm going to call—again, this is in hindsight, I wish I could go do it, but I can't—'Let me call some people. Let me call my family. Let me call my mother. Let me call my sponsors. Let me call my foundation and tell them what I'm going to do, and I'll be right there.' I wish I could do that. But I can't."

* Even so, it could not help but become personal, especially considering that Tygart received numerous death threats during the Armstrong case. "The worst was, putting a bullet in my head," he told *60 Minutes Sports*.

USADA, not the media, and certainly not Lance—was providing them.

That was when our book came out.

In a heartbeat my life turned into a crazy tumble of cameras, microphones, and interviewers, everybody urgently wanting to know about me, about what I had to say, about why I came forward now. It felt strange, after so much time in exile, to be in the middle of the hurricane again.

If you happened to see me on TV, you know I'm not the greatest interviewee on the planet. Truth is, I was never comfortable in the spotlight when I was a rider, and not much has changed on that front. I'm not the kind of guy who can deliver a clever line over and over again like an actor. But I did my best to tell the truth.

I caused a bit of a stir the morning the book came out while talking with Matt Lauer on *The Today Show*. Lauer was pointing out that Armstrong and the UCI vehemently denied that he'd doped, and I responded by saying, "It doesn't surprise me that they deny it; I denied it for years. After a while you get pretty good at it. I've lied to you before, straight to your face." Lauer gave a surprised blink, and the Twittersphere flared with disbelief – *Hamilton admits to lying!* Judging by the reaction, I'm sure it wasn't the smartest PR move in the world, but I was glad I said it, because it shows what this story is really about: confronting the truth, especially about myself. Being open, even when it's uncomfortable. *Especially* when it's uncomfortable.

After a few days in the media circus, I escaped to Marblehead, my childhood home. The hugs I got from my mom and dad were like no embrace I'd ever gotten: big, long, hard hugs, like I'd just returned from an expedition to Mount Everest. We didn't say much. We just sat looking at each other, feeling the world change underneath our feet.

Nearly as fulfilling were the messages I got from friends and family who were reading the book. In the space of a few days, I got hundreds of emails, texts, letters, Facebook and Twitter messages; nearly every one was warm and kind—though I certainly didn't blame the handful who weren't ready to forgive me yet, and who wanted to hold my feet to the fire, and wondered why I didn't have the guts to tell the truth the first time. But all in all, reading those messages made me realize how much the secret had been a wall between me and my friends, and made me grateful for having the chance for a fresh start.

I'd been worried that my old teammates would hate me for writing a book; that they would feel I'd broken some unwritten rule or forced them into the limelight when they weren't ready to be there. But the teammates I communicated with were nice about it (Frankie Andreu posted a funny photo of himself reading *The Secret Race* with his fingers pressed to his lips, as if he were shocked); Floyd and I exchanged friendly text messages; I also heard from a number of younger riders who appreciated my openness. The truth was, some of them were shocked, especially the teammates from later years. They knew the general picture, but they'd never heard all the gory details. I guess that was a measure of how crazy and dysfunctional a time it was: you can ride next to someone, live with them, share meals with them, but you have to wait ten years to find out the truth about what was happening behind closed doors.

The book helped trigger others to start talking: Michel Rieu, scientific advisor to the French testing lab AFLD, told *Le Monde* that Lance was warned before tests. My old teammate Jonathan Vaughters started talking as well. At one point, on a cycling forum, he mentioned that several members of his Garmin team, including Christian Vande Velde, Dave Zabriskie, and Tom Danielson, had doped earlier in their careers, effectively outing those riders. Whether it was an accident or a more calculated maneuver was unclear, but the larger point was, it didn't really matter. The avalanche was underway.

The biggest question, of course, was when USADA would release its "reasoned decision", which was standard procedure in doping cases such as this. Normally, it's a measured, legalistic document that sums up the evidence and logic behind the USADA decision and penalty. In Lance's case, however, it was clear that this was going to be bigger. The question was, what would it contain?

The days leading up to the decision's October release were like one long drumroll. One by one, the riders who had cooperated with the investigation issued public statements that essentially said yep, they'd doped. Of those, George Hincapie's confession was the biggest deal, since he'd always been perceived as closest to Lance, the loyal soldier, and had never been linked to any doping. But in a few sentences, that all changed.

"*Early in my professional career, it became clear to me that, given the widespread use of performance enhancing drugs by cyclists at the top of the profession, it was not possible to compete at the highest level without them. I deeply regret that choice and sincerely apologize to my family, teammates and fans."*

I read those statements, and I felt for George and the rest of the guys. I knew how hard it was to write those words, and to look into the faces of family and friends who'd believed, and tell the truth. I was glad we could all do it together, as a group, since that was the only way it could happen: everybody taking the leap at once. Omertà in reverse.

On the afternoon of October 10, USADA released its reasoned decision. Everyone had presumed it would be a large document, and everyone was wrong: it was gigantic. One thousand pages of devastating evidence; a sledge-hammer of carefully annotated proof that Armstrong was a key player in "the most sophisticated, professionalized, and successful doping program sport has ever seen". There's far too much key information to recount fully, but here's the big picture:

- Testimony from 26 people, including 11 teammates.
- Numerous accounts of Lance using blood transfusions, EPO, human growth hormone, cortisone, and testosterone.
- Detailed accounts dating from 1998, when Lance used saline infusions to dilute his blood and evade a test at the World Championships.
- Financial records detailing more than $1 million in payments from Lance to Dr. Ferrari, including after Ferrari's conviction in 2004, when Lance had publicly stated they were no longer working together.

- Numerous accounts of Lance bullying and threatening people to keep the secret quiet.
- Scientific analysis of Lance's blood during his 2009-10 comeback that showed he had blood doped.

For me, though, the most compelling parts weren't the evidence so much as the affidavits from my former teammates:

Dave Zabriskie told about his rough background—how his father had a drug problem that drove young Dave into the sport and gave him a deep aversion to drugs of all kinds. How Dave had ridden clean as he rose through the national team and was signed to Postal in 2001. How Dave stated he was then pressured to use EPO and testosterone by Bruyneel, who provided it one afternoon at a Girona cafe. Worried, Dave asked questions: would it change his body? Would he be able to have children? After using EPO for the first time, Dave returned to his apartment and had an emotional breakdown.

Levi Leipheimer told how Bruyneel and del Moral helped perfect his regimen so he would peak at big races. How, when Levi returned to the Discovery team in 2007, he asked Bruyneel if the team was organizing a blood doping program for the Tour de France; Bruyneel's reply: "You're a pro, you should do it on your own." How, two years later, when Levi discussed the possibility of using a new drug being discussed in the media, Lance replied, "You know I'm always down for it." And how, in the fall of 2010, after Levi testified before the grand jury, Lance sent a threatening text to Levi's wife that read, "Run, don't walk."

There was Christian Vande Velde telling how Kristin Armstrong wrapped cortisone pills in foil and distributed them to the team at the 1998 World Championships; how he'd delivered cortisone to Lance during a stage of the 1998 Vuelta to help him finish a stage; how he was summoned to Lance's apartment, where Lance told him that "if I wanted to continue to ride for the Postal Service team I would have to use what Dr. Ferrari had been telling me to use and follow Dr. Ferrari's program to the letter."

USADA's reasoned decision changed the landscape, allowing millions of people to see the truth for themselves. Poetically enough, this was also when we got to see the truth about Pat McQuaid and the leaders of the UCI. When reporters asked about the USADA report, McQuaid attempted to squirm away from his earlier support of Lance, saying—in a complete 180—that Lance "deserves to be forgotten by cycling." But then McQuaid kept talking, adamantly denying that the donations the UCI had received from Armstrong were improper, and avoiding any responsibility for cycling's doping problem. Then he talked about Floyd and me, attacking Floyd for speaking out and attacking me for writing the book. He referred to us as "scumbags," and said, "All they have done is damage the sport."

I don't get mad very often. But when the president of the UCI—the organization that had presided over omertà and protected Lance for all these years for its own enrichment—attacks people for telling the truth, I can't help but speak out. I sat down at my computer and typed out a statement:

"Pat McQuaid's comments expose the hypocrisy of his

leadership and demonstrate why he is incapable of any meaningful change," I wrote. "Instead of seizing an opportunity to instill hope for the next generation of cyclists, he continues to point fingers, shift blame and attack those who speak out, tactics that are no longer effective. Pat McQuaid has no place in cycling.'"*

The UCI might have kept its blinders on, but others did not. Particularly the companies who'd stood loyally beside Lance through all the controversy. In a few stunning hours after the reasoned decision was released, they'd all vanished—Nike, Oakley, Trek, Anheuser-Busch, and the rest—in a $75 million cloud of smoke. While it was the right thing to do, I found the speed of their departure disturbing. After all, these were the same companies that used all their power to build the Armstrong myth, ignoring years of legitimate doubts about his performance, to make him and themselves millions of dollars.

But the avalanche was just beginning. SCA Insurance, which had underwritten his bonuses, geared up to file a lawsuit for $12 million; the *Sunday Times* of London

---

* In the wake of the USADA report, the UCI attempted a familiar move: they appointed a three-person commission to look into the problem and produce a report. In an unusually candid response, USADA announced "grave concerns" about the UCI's commitment to a full investigation, and said that they would reject the commission and renew the call for a truth and reconciliation period. In late January, the UCI caved, abandoning the commission.

In January 2013, after repeatedly denying that the UCI had informed Armstrong of his suspicious drug tests, former UCI president Hein Verbruggen admitted that his organization had warned certain riders, including Armstrong, about their blood values. Verbruggen continued to deny any

began preparing to fight to claw back their $1 million. Lance was also on the hook for all the prize money he'd won since 1998. Not to mention the big one: the Qi Tam whistleblower lawsuit brought by Floyd Landis, alleging that Tailwind Sports (whose ownership included Lance, Bill Stapleton, Thom Weisel, and Johan Bruyneel) had defrauded the U.S. Postal Service by violating the no-doping clause in their contract, and which carried a total potential liability of $90 million. All in all, potential losses added up to around $100 million.

As I watched the avalanche fall, my emotions were mixed. I felt a massive sense of relief that the secret was coming out, and that people would have the chance to see the truth and make up their own minds. I felt happy for all those who'd been victimized by Lance's bullying, and sorry for clean riders who'd had to leave the sport. Part of me also felt sorry for Lance. I knew what it was like to have everything taken away, to be thrown into the wilderness. I knew the pain of public humiliation. And I couldn't help but wonder what he would do to try to recover, to strike back.

responsibility for the era's rampant doping, telling the Dutch magazine *De Muur*, "I don't understand the whole fuss at all. If you test someone 215 times and he is always negative, then the problem is in the test itself. Well, I'm not responsible."

In addition, it turned out that Verbruggen had maintained a personal investment account with Postal team owner Thom Weisel during the Armstrong era, according to the *Wall Street Journal*. Verbruggen again denied any impropriety, but as USADA president Tygart put it, "To have the head of the sport, who's responsible for enforcing anti-doping rules, in business with the owner of the team that won seven straight Tours de France in violation of those rules—it certainly stinks to high heaven, particularly now, given what's been exposed that happened under his watch."

In November, Dan and I got some good news: *The Secret Race* had been nominated for Britain's William Hill Sports Book of the Year Award. We found ourselves at the ceremony, in Waterstone's bookstore on Piccadilly. The place was packed with the royalty of the British sportswriting world; all around us were giant posters of the previous winners (including, in 2000, Lance's memoir *It's Not About the Bike*). When the judges announced that we'd won, we couldn't quite absorb it.

It was only later, after the champagne toasts, that I realized something. Since almost all of my racing results had been stripped from the record books, this award was now the only clean victory I'd won in a long while.

The photo on Twitter showed Lance reclining on a massive sectional couch in his Austin home beneath seven framed yellow jerseys. Beneath it he'd written, "Back in Austin and just layin' around."

It looked like precisely what it was: a middle finger to the world. Thing was, he wasn't layin' around, but doing the opposite: huddling with his brain trust, plotting his next move, trying to figure out how he might get his ban reduced. I'd heard he was calling journalists and friends, lobbying his case, venting his anger, which flowed from his belief that he'd been treated unfairly by USADA. Why had the others only gotten a six-month ban, and he got a lifetime ban? Why had he been singled out?

In late fall, Lance started pushing his attorneys to arrange a meeting with Tygart. In mid-December he flew to Denver, and the two met in a conference room near the airport. According to *Wall Street Journal*'s account of the meeting, Lance talked openly about his doping. He complained about being singled out, and pointed out that the NFL and other sports were rife with cheating. Tygart was unmoved, reminding Lance that he'd already had a chance to come clean, that he stood accused of offenses far beyond doping, including coverups, threats, and conspiracy to conceal fraud. Tygart told Lance that the best he could hope for was to cooperate fully, under oath, and he would have a chance to get his ban reduced to eight years.

"You don't hold the keys to my redemption," Armstrong said, according to the story. "There's only one person who holds the keys to my redemption, and that's me." And then he walked out.

After that, I think it was only a matter of time before Lance did something big. He can't help it; it's the way he's wired. He gets pissed, and he needs to respond. He needs to *shut people up*, and take control of the situation. He has to prove to the world that he was still Lance Armstrong.

So he called Oprah.

Afterward, commentators spoke about how calculated this decision was, how it must have been part of some larger master comeback plan. To my thinking, however, it was the opposite: an instinctive, emotional roll of the dice. Lance made the decision to call Oprah in the same way he made the decision in 1999 to use Motoman, or to attack Pantani on Mont Ventoux in 2000, or any of the million other aggressive moves Lance has made over the years. Big risk, big return—or so he hoped.

A few days before the interview, Lance started making

apologies. He reached out to the LeMonds, Floyd, Emma; he apologized to the staff of Livestrong. I was told he sent me an apologetic email, but I never received it. The Andreus spoke with him, but kept the details private. The rest, including Floyd and the LeMonds, chose not to speak to Lance, and instead expressed incredulity—how could he attack them for years and then try to make it up with a phone call on the eve of talking to Oprah?

I was in New York the night of the interview, and it felt like a weird class reunion: Vaughters was in the same hotel, in the room exactly above mine and Lindsay's; Betsy Andreu was down the street; Floyd a few miles away in Connecticut. All around the world, people were asking the same question: would Lance really come clean? Would he be contrite? Oprah kicked off with a bang, a series of yes/no questions.

Oprah: Did you ever take banned substances to enhance your cycling performance?
Lance: Yes.
O: Was one of those banned substances EPO?
L: Yes.
O: Did you ever blood dope or use blood transfusions to enhance your cycling performance?
L: Yes.
O: Did you ever use any other banned substances such as testosterone, cortisone or human growth hormone?
L: Yes.
O: In all seven of your Tour de France victories, did you ever take banned substances or blood dope?
L: Yes.

It was just five words. Five matter-of-fact nods. But to me, those five words were like land mines going off one by one, detonating that world of lies that had been built so carefully, that had stood for so many years. All the fighting, all the win-at-all-costs scheming, all the lying and threatening and bullying—that insane world I'd lived inside, and escaped—it suddenly vanished. All that was left was Lance, sitting in a chair, looking scared. Looking small. Looking human.

Yes.

Most people focused on how calculating and hesitant Lance seemed. They noted how smoothly he offered to throw his loyal supporters at the UCI under the bus ("I'm not a big fan of the UCI," he said at a couple points). They focused on how un-contrite and cocky he seemed, particularly when he tried to joke about his attacks on Betsy Andreu. "I called you crazy, I called you a bitch," he said, speaking directly to Betsy. "I called you all those things, but I never called you fat." More important—and more curiously—he resisted confirming her sworn account of the hospital room incident from 1996, when she and others testified Armstrong admitted to doctors that he'd used performance-enhancing drugs. *

In addition, Lance made the dubious claim to have

---

* Why would Armstrong not admit the truth about the hospital room, when he was admitting so much? Two possibilities: 1) he was protecting those who had testified under oath that it had not happened; 2) he was simply stubborn. Either way, it did not go over well with Betsy Andreu. "You owed it to me, Lance, and you dropped the ball," she said to CNN, her voice filling with raw emotion. "After what you've done to me, what you've done to my family, and you couldn't own up to it. And now we're supposed to believe you?"

ridden his 2009–10 comeback clean (tests showed there was less than a one in a million chance of his blood profile happening naturally),* and also that he had not encouraged doping on the Postal team. (I nearly laughed out loud at that one; I'd bet the other Posties did too.) He also denied a more recent *60 Minutes Sports* report that his representatives had attempted to offer USADA a six-figure "gift" in 2004.†

Oprah did a good job. She'd clearly done her homework, and she reacted to many of Lance's answers with a mix of exasperation and disbelief. Watching their tense exchanges felt like watching the most unsuccessful therapy session in history, a mix of evasions, calculations, and outright lies, all of it threaded through with an almost scary lack of empathy. A real confession (and after the last couple years, I count myself as something of an expert) depends on being 100 percent open, showing emotion, and being truly, deeply sorry. They're not about what you do. They're about what you feel,

---

* The possible logic behind Armstrong's tactic: if he managed to persuade USADA that he'd stopped doping in 2005, they could potentially reduce his lifetime ban to eight years, meaning he could come back to WADA-sanctioned sports in 2013. Given that Armstrong had, as of February 2013, shown no signs of cooperating with USADA's investigation, this appears highly unlikely.

† Former USADA president Terry Madden later confirmed that one of Armstrong's "closest representatives" had offered USADA a "donation" in the range of $250,000 in 2004, and that USADA had reacted swiftly. "Travis [Tygart's] office was about a five-second walk from mine," Madden told ESPN. "He informed me, and we immediately rejected the idea. I told him to go back and call the representative and inform him that based on our ethics, we could not accept a donation from anyone we were testing [for performance-enhancing drugs and techniques] or would test in the future."

and now the world got to see what some of us have known for a long time: Lance is not so good at feeling.

Still, there were moments of authenticity, like when Oprah showed a clip of him denying doping under oath in 2005, and asked Lance what he thought about this past version of himself.

"That defiance, that attitude, that arrogance," he said, with a disgusted shake of the head. "You cannot deny it. You watch that clip and that's an arrogant person. Look at that, I say, look at that arrogant prick. I say that today. It's not good."

I found myself feeling a tug of sympathy for the guy. I knew how hard it was for him to say those words. While by normal standards Lance seemed un-contrite, I was struck by the fact that, for Lance, this qualified as groveling. He said phrases I'd never heard him say, like "I'm sorry," and "I apologize." He looked shaken, brittle, haggard.

Instantly, the reviews flowed in, and they were not favorable. Even Lance's former cheerleaders like Rick Reilly and Buzz Bissinger were leading the torch-and-pitchfork mob. Reilly, who'd called for a national Wear Yellow campaign to support Lance in August, when USADA had stripped his Tour de France titles, now compared Lance's affect to that of "a hit man testifying before Congress." Bissinger, who'd defended Lance in an August cover story for *Newsweek*, now called him, "an immoral, manipulative liar who doesn't deserve a second of anyone's time." The anti-doping authorities were about as friendly.

"What [Armstrong] is doing is for his own personal

gratification," said WADA director David Howman. "He's welcome to do that, no one is going to criticize that component, but if anyone thinks that in his wildest dreams that it is going to have any effect on his life ban then they are in the same fairyland."

Things got even worse for Lance two weeks later, when it was revealed that federal officials were actively pursuing a criminal investigation against him for witness tampering, obstruction, and intimidation. I'd guess that some of this stems from his June 2011 attempt to intimidate me in Aspen, and to be honest, I'm not sure how I feel about it. On one hand, he did say he was going to tear me apart on the witness stand, and make my life "a living fucking hell", and I don't think anybody should be above the law. On the other hand, I feel some empathy for Lance, and I don't want to see him go to prison. At some point, enough is enough.

Of all the things we learned in the Oprah interview, I was most glad to hear Lance say that he was in therapy. In my opinion, that's what it takes: a lot of hard work, time, and real reflection. All of us who've confessed have gone through dark times; most of us have suffered from some form of depression; I'm sure Lance is not immune to this. I hope he has the friends and family to support him.

Will Lance change? I have no idea, except to say that it's clear he has taken the first step by telling the truth, albeit in partial form. I do know that because the lie is so big and so vast, the truth can only emerge in stages. It's not like he can flip a switch and suddenly be 100 percent transparent; it's more like excavating a buried city. It takes a lot of shovelwork, time, and effort, and most of all the willingness to endure the pain. It's not pretty. But I can say that it is worthwhile.

I hear the question all the time, in interviews, on the sidewalk, in coffee shops: Can the sport recover? I say that on one hand, the sport *is* recovering: much progress has been made since the Wild West days of my era. On the other, it's clear that if the progress is going to continue, there are five things that have to happen:

1 Convene a truth and reconciliation commission where, for a limited amount of time, all riders can come forward and tell the whole truth about their careers without fear of reprisal or penalty. Without trust, nothing will happen.*

2 Replace the UCI with an entirely new set of leaders who are 100 percent committed to doing whatever it takes to support clean sport.

3 Enlist law-enforcement officials to help police the sport and provide enforcement, and increase international cooperation to help track down PED supply lines and uncover illicit financial networks.

---

* In December, USADA drafted an eight-point proposal on how a truth and reconciliation commission might proceed. The letter suggested that the commission be run by WADA, which would provide a month-long amnesty window, during which riders, support staff, and team ownership could come forward. Those who provided full and complete written statements about their own doping and knowledge of others would be eligible for amnesty. They would also sign an agreement that any further anti-doping violation would be punished with a lifetime ban from the sport.

4   Move away from the sponsorship model of teams (where teams are bankrolled by corporations) and toward a more stable private-ownership model, as in the NFL or major league baseball. The problem with sponsors is that they require immediate return on their investment, creating a win-at-all-costs ethos that trickles down through management to riders. The more stable the team, the less pressure to dope.

5   Keep improving the biological passport which, like any system, has its loopholes that can be exploited, and make sure it's administrated and enforced by an independent entity.

Deep change happens slowly, and nowhere is this more true than in our sport. The avalanche might have come, but omertà does not disappear overnight—far from it. In recent months, we've seen several riders and coaches lose their jobs simply for telling the truth about their pasts. We should be doing the opposite: encouraging confession and truth, not burying it and following the old pattern of denying, avoiding, and pretending everything is fine, and criticizing anyone who speaks out.

That said, there are a few hopeful signs, such as Change Cycling Now, a grassroots effort that's a *Who's Who* of anti-doping activists like Paul Kimmage, David Walsh, and Greg LeMond (who volunteered himself as an interim leader for the UCI). My old teammate Scott Mercier has been speaking up for clean cycling as well, even volunteering to coach at Colorado Mesa University when the previous coach was fired after he admitted to doping riders. It's far too early to say if these efforts will lead to long-term success, but they're proof that change can happen, and they're also proof that cycling, unlike so many other sports, is attempting to confront the problem, not merely hiding from it (yep, NFL, NBA and major league baseball, I'm talking about you).

As for me, I don't ride my bike much anymore, mostly using it to run errands around town. For exercise, I prefer to go hiking or jogging, because the speed suits both Lindsay and me, and because we can bring Tanker along. We head out from our house and we can be high in the hills around Mount Sentinel in a few minutes, getting lost, and letting Tanker chase after chipmunks. But he's not the only one searching for something. I am, too: I'm looking for pieces of wood.

Here's my last confession: I'm addicted to woodworking. I know, it sounds like an old man's hobby, but I love it. So when we're out hiking, I'll pick up armfuls of branches and deadfall, carry them home, and start whittling, cutting, carving. The guys at the local Ace Hardware store get excited when they see me come in the door: they know I'm going to leave with some new tools. I probably have twenty different projects I've started—a chair, a small table, salad forks—and I've barely finished any of them. But it's not the finishing I like; it's the doing. I love the process of seeing some form hidden inside and trying to bring that out.

The other day Lindsay and I drove just over the border into Idaho, to a place called the Jerry Johnson Hot Springs where there had been a big fire. What had once been a beautiful cedar forest was now a sad moonscape of charred stumps. We wandered around, and pulled a few pieces out of the rubble, including one small stump. It looked ruined. But underneath, when I carved away the blackness, I saw the fire had made the wood harder, better.

I carried the stump home, took it to the garage, and started working on it. I like the smell, the leathery feel of it; I like touching the circles of those age-rings. I guess part of me likes to hope that I'm like that piece of wood: charred and damaged, but also stronger, shaping myself into some new purpose that only time will reveal.

Thanks for reading.

Tyler Hamilton
Missoula, Montana
February 2013

Acknowledgments

TYLER HAMILTON:

This book would not exist without Daniel Coyle. What started with a simple email has grown into a deep friendship. It is such a huge relief to have this book completed, but I will miss our sometimes painful, sometimes fun, always interesting ten-hour-long Skype sessions. (Can we still do that, by the way?) In all seriousness, thank you, Dan.

I want to thank Andy Ward and the crew at Random House for believing in this project early on, and for the hard work and dedication they showed under unique circumstances.

To David Black (aka Bull Dog): you are my first, best, and last literary agent. Thank you so much and GO RED SOX!!!

A special thanks to Melinda Travis for always having my back through thick and thin.

A gigantic, heartfelt thanks to my extraordinary

parents, Lorna and Bill, who have shown me the true meaning of grace and humility. You taught me that the truth will set me free and you were right. My eyes are open and the weight has been lifted. I could not have asked for a better support system. An equally heartfelt thanks to my brother and sister, Geoff and Jenn: thanks for your immense support and encouragement during the process of writing the book. The many ups and downs of my career have been a challenge for our family, but we would not have gotten through it without your unconditional love and support. You guys are the best.

Thanks to Haven Parchinski for your lasting friendship, to Steve Pucci for believing, to Phil Peck for your wisdom, to Chris Manderson for your warmth and generosity, to Dr. Charles Welch for your understanding and guidance, and especially to Robert Frost, Erich Kaiter, Patrick Brown, Jill Alfond, Matty O'Keefe, and Guy Cherp for your special friendships.

Thanks to each and every one of my old teammates on Montgomery, U.S. Postal Service, CSC, Phonak, and Rock Racing for all the good times we shared that none of us will ever forget.

A special shout-out to Jim "Capo" Capra for being a solid rock. You took the handlebars of my business when I could no longer steer it. Without you there would be no Tyler Hamilton Training LLC.

Jimmy Huega, may you rest in peace. My life is better because you were a part of it.

To Cecco, Anna, Anzano, and Stefano, my European family, *grazie mille*.

Thanks to Tanker for always being underfoot.

And finally, to my wonderful wife, Lindsay: thank you for your willingness, bravery, and enthusiasm for taking this journey into my past—and also for the love and companionship you bring to the life we're building together. You make all good things possible.

DANIEL COYLE:

I would like to thank Lindsay Hamilton, Mike Paterniti, Tom Kizzia, Mary Turner, Mark Bryant, John Giuggio, Paul Cox, Trent MacNamara, Kaela Myers, Allison Hemphill, Jim Capra, Robert Frost, Jim Aikman, Ken Wohlrob, Kim Hovey, Cindy Murray, Benjamin Dreyer, Steve Messina, Bill Adams, Jennifer Hershey, and Libby McGuire. I'd also like to express my gratitude for the work of David Walsh, Pierre Ballester, and Paul Kimmage. I'd especially like to thank my terrific agent, David Black, my brilliant editor, Andy Ward, and my brother, Maurice Coyle, whose impact on this book (and every other one I write) is immeasurable. I'd like to thank my parents, Maurice and Agnes; my brother, Jon; my children, Aidan, Katie, Lia, and Zoe; and my wife, Jen, who makes everything go. Above all, I'd like to thank Tyler Hamilton for his honesty, his courage, and his friendship.

Further Reading

The (Honest) Truth About Dishonesty, by Dan Ariely
Rough Ride, by Paul Kimmage
Racing Through the Dark, by David Millar
The Death of Marco Pantani, by Matt Rendell
Riis: Stages of Light and Dark, by Bjarne Riis
Breaking the Chain, by Willy Voet
From Lance to Landis, by David Walsh
Bad Blood, by Jeremy Whittle
The Crooked Path to Victory, by Les Woodland
"The Effect of EPO on Performance: Who Wouldn't Want to Use It?" by Dr. Ross Tucker: *http://www.sportsscientists.com/2007/11/effect-of-epo-on-performance-who.html*
Interview with Dr. Michael Ashenden on Armstrong's likely EPO use during the 1999 Tour de France: *http://nyvelocity.com/content/interviews/2009/michael-ashenden*
Court transcript from Armstrong's 2005 lawsuit against

former assistant Mike Anderson: *http://alt.coxnewsweb.com/statesman/sports/040105_lance.pdf*

Transcript of Lance Armstrong's sworn testimony in the 2005 SCA Promotions arbitration case: *http://www.scribd.com/doc/31833754/Lance-Armstrong-Testimony*

In addition, videos of Armstrong's SCA testimony can be found at *http://nyvelocity.com/content/features/2011/armstrong-sca-deposition-videos*